MIND OVER GUT

How Self-Hypnosis and Hypnotherapy Can Help Manage IBS Symptoms, Improve Gut Health, and Enhance the Gut-Brain Connection

- Linda Baker -

Table of Contents

Acknowledgements

First and foremost, I'm so grateful to all the brave souls living with Irritable Bowel Syndrome (IBS) who've opened up to me about their journeys. Your stories of courage and resilience are the heart of this book, and I'm deeply touched by your honesty and strength. A huge shoutout to the healthcare heroes, especially those wizards in gastroenterology and hypnotherapy, for their priceless insights. Your commitment to solving the IBS puzzle brings so much hope to many.

Big thanks to the support groups and online communities out there – you're amazing! You offer a comforting space for people to connect, share stories, and find a sense of belonging. You're making a world of difference in the lives of those grappling with IBS.

To my family and friends, you are my rock! Your constant support, belief in my work, and the pep talks have been the wind beneath my wings. And to my peers in physical education, thank you for standing by me and valuing the whole picture of health, both physical and mental.

A round of applause for the editors, publishers, and everyone who played a part in bringing this book to life. Your skills and dedication helped shape this into a tool that I believe will transform many lives. Lastly, if you've ever felt isolated in your struggle with IBS, remember this book is for you. It's a reminder that hope, relief, and a supportive community are always within reach. Your experiences have inspired this journey of healing and exploration.

Thank you all for being part of this incredible journey. Together, let's spread the word that better days are ahead, and help is always at hand! I've just completed week five of my hypnotherapy journey, and guess what? Last night, I enjoyed fish with garlic, honey, and mustard in my salad dressing, and I felt absolutely fine – no symptoms at all! Gradually, I plan to reintroduce more FODMAP foods into my diet. This experience has been incredibly enlightening, helping me not only understand my issues better but also manage them effectively.

"Just one week into my self-hypnosis journey, I've already introduced around 10 new foods to my diet. Now, after completing the week-long program, I'm ecstatic to share that I've completely moved away from the low FODMAP diet. I'm enjoying garlic, onions, dairy, and even dining out! This experience feels like magic, yet I'm fascinated by its scientific basis."

Introduction

Picture this: You're on a path that's as unpredictable as the weather, a path shared by millions worldwide. This is the journey of living with Irritable Bowel Syndrome, a journey I've walked alongside many. Each person carries their unique story of symptoms that sway like a pendulum – abdominal pain, bloating, a seesaw of bowel habits from constipation to diarrhea, and sometimes, an unpredictable mix of both. These are not just symptoms; they're the threads that weave through every aspect of life, tangling with emotional and mental well-being.

Let me tell you about the unpredictability of IBS.

You wake up each morning, unsure if the day will be smooth sailing or if you'll be navigating through a storm of discomfort. It's like planning a picnic under clear skies, only to have an unexpected downpour. This constant uncertainty can cloud over daily routines, work commitments, and even the simplest joys of social gatherings. It's not just about managing symptoms; it's about managing life itself, often under the watchful eyes of misunderstanding.

In the world of IBS, the struggle often wears an invisible cloak. Without outward signs, garnering understanding and empathy becomes a challenge in itself. I've seen the loneliness and frustration this invisibility brings, making the IBS journey a solitary one for many. And then there's the never-ending detective work – figuring out what triggers the symptoms. It could be a certain food, stress, or something as unpredictable as a change in weather. This vigilant search, while well-intentioned, can sometimes feel like chasing shadows, only adding to the complexity of IBS.

The road to finding relief is as unique as the condition itself. No two stories of IBS are the same, which means what brings relief to one may not work for another. This individuality turns the quest for comfort into a winding journey of exploration – sometimes hopeful, sometimes disheartening. The absence of a universal solution, a magic key to unlock relief, often leaves many in a loop of trial and error.

But here's the silver lining in this intricate journey. Recognizing the full spectrum of IBS – understanding that it's more than a list of symptoms, that it's a dance of physical, emotional, and psychological elements – is the first step towards empowerment. It's about embracing the journey not just as a physical challenge but as an integral part of your life's narrative. This is where hypnotherapy steps in, like a trusted friend, offering not just a balm for the symptoms but a harmonious melody for the mind and body.

Remember, you're not treading this path alone.

As I share my own experiences and insights, I hope to walk with you, lending a friendly voice to guide you through the ups and downs. Hypnotherapy, a tool I've found invaluable, can be a transformative ally in your IBS story. It's not just about easing the symptoms; it's about finding a rhythm in the chaos, a sense of control amidst the unpredictable. It's about learning to listen to your body and mind, harmonizing them in a way that brings relief and a newfound sense of empowerment.

This journey with IBS is a personal odyssey that touches every facet of your life. But within this odyssey lies a story of resilience, strength, and hope. With each step, you learn, you adapt, and you grow. Hypnotherapy can be that gentle guide, helping you navigate the rough waters, bringing you closer to calm shores.

So, as you continue on this path, remember that every challenge is a stepping stone towards understanding yourself better. Each day is an opportunity to embrace your health journey, not just as a series of symptoms to be managed, but as a holistic experience that shapes your story.

In "Mind Over Gut," we delve deeper into this narrative. The book begins by laying the foundation – understanding IBS, its diverse symptoms, and the daily challenges it poses. It then guides you through the fascinating science behind hypnosis, unraveling how it effectively manages IBS.

The book arms you with practical hypnotherapy techniques, enriches you with real-life success stories, and guides you in weaving these practices into your daily life for a more holistic approach to managing IBS. As we turn the pages, you'll encounter inspiring tales of resilience and transformation, stories that illuminate the path towards regaining control over your body's responses. It's about fostering a sense of well-being and resilience, a journey where you're the pilot, steering towards calmer waters. This book is crafted to be your companion, guiding you through each step with empathy and understanding.

Further, "Mind Over Gut" addresses the common questions and doubts that may cloud your mind about hypnotherapy. It's natural to have concerns, to wonder about the unknown. This book seeks to dispel myths and shed light on the holistic nature of managing IBS through hypnotherapy. It's an exploration of how this approach goes beyond mere symptom management, empowering you to embrace a life where IBS doesn't dictate your story.

Chapter 1: Understanding IBS

Irritable Bowel Syndrome (IBS) is a common gastrointestinal disorder that significantly impacts the lives of millions worldwide. This condition is characterized by a complex interplay of symptoms, including abdominal pain, bloating, and changes in bowel habits, that deeply affect individua' quality of life. It is a multifaceted disorder, as it encompasses a range of symptoms and experiences that can vary greatly from person to person. This variability underscores the importance of a nuanced approach to diagnosis and management, reflecting the individual nature of the condition.

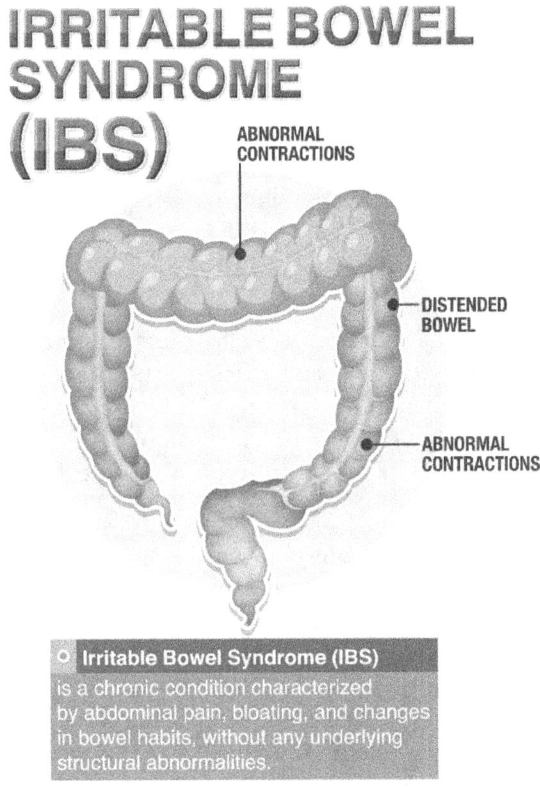

The predominant symptoms determine the classification of IBS into three main types: IBS-C, IBS-D, and IBS-M or IBS-A.

For instance, IBS-C is characterized by chronic constipation, making bowel movements infrequent or difficult, often accompanied by abdominal pain, bloating, and a sense of incomplete evacuation even after a bowel movement. Unlike ordinary constipation, it involves a dysregulation of the gut-brain axis which leads to alterations in bowel motility and sensitivity, contributing to the symptoms experienced. Furthermore, IBS-C is characterized by a multifactorial pathophysiology that includes genetic predispositions, low-grade inflammation of the gut, altered gut microbiota, and increased intestinal permeability, often referred to as "leaky gut."

On the other end of the spectrum, IBS-D is marked by its hallmark symptom of recurrent, loose, or watery stools, which is often paired with an urgent need to use the bathroom, and the individuals with IBS-D typically experience abdominal pain and discomfort, which can significantly disrupt daily activities and decrease the quality of life. Its underlying mechanisms involve a complex interplay between gut motility, sensitivity, and the microbiome. Abnormalities in the gastrointestinal tract's movement may lead to accelerated bowel transit times, contributing to the diarrhea predominant nature of this subtype. Additionally, a heightened sensitivity to gut movements and the presence of certain foods can worsen symptoms, making dietary management a key component of treatment. Furthermore, emerging research highlights the role of the gut microbiota in IBS-D, suggesting that imbalances in these microbial communities may influence the condition's pathophysiology.

IBS-M/A, as the name suggests, presents a particularly challenging condition where individuals experience a volatile mixture of both constipation (IBS-C) and diarrhea (IBS-D) symptoms. This variant of IBS is characterized by unforeseeable and often fluctuating patterns of bowel movements, where patients may endure periods of hard, difficult-to-pass stools followed by phases of loose or watery stools. The transition between these extremes can be rapid, adding a layer of complexity to daily life and symptom management.

Diagnosing the Irritable Bowel Syndrome presents its own set of challenges, primarily due to the absence of a definitive test. The Rome IV criteria focus on recurrent abdominal pain for at least one day a week in the last three months, associated with two or more factors: related to defecation, associated with a change in the frequency of stool, or associated with a change in the form (appearance) of stool. The reliance on symptom-based criteria emphasizes the importance of a thorough medical history and patient-doctor communication in diagnosing IBS, highlighting the challenges in distinguishing it from other gastrointestinal disorders with similar symptoms.

The condition's hallmark symptoms, including alterations in gut motility, visceral hypersensitivity, and the impact of microbiota dysbiosis and inflammation, paint a picture of a disorder that is as multifaceted in its underpinnings as it is in its manifestations.

Gut motility refers to the movements of the digestive system that propel contents through the gastrointestinal tract. In IBS, these movements can become dysregulated, leading either to accelerated transit times, seen in IBS with diarrhea (IBS-D), or slowed processes, observed in IBS with constipation (IBS-C). This dysregulation can result from a variety of factors, including abnormalities in the nervous system that controls gut movements or changes in the levels of neurotransmitters and hormones that regulate gut function. The result is a spectrum of symptoms that directly impact an individual's quality of life, from urgent bowel movements to painful bloating and constipation.

Another critical piece of the IBS puzzle is visceral hypersensitivity, or an increased sensitivity to pain and discomfort within the gut. This phenomenon means that sensations that might not bother others, such as the stretching of the gut wall during normal digestion, can cause significant pain or discomfort in individuals with IBS.

In the upcoming chapters we will focus on the role of the gut microbiota and inflammation in IBS, which highlights the complex interplay between our bodies and the microscopic organisms that reside within us. Research has shown that individuals with IBS often exhibit an imbalance in the composition of the gut microbiota. This can contribute to symptoms through several mechanisms, including the production of gas and other metabolites that can irritate the gut lining, modulation of gut motility, and interaction with the immune system, potentially leading to low-grade inflammation. Such inflammation, in turn, can exacerbate visceral hypersensitivity and further disrupt gut motility, creating a cycle of discomfort and distress. However, before we explore these interactions and their implications, it's essential to lay the groundwork by understanding the common remedies available for IBS. This foundational knowledge will equip us with the necessary context to appreciate the significance of gut health and its impact on IBS management, setting the stage for a deeper investigation into targeted strategies that address the root causes of this condition.

Common Remedies

The condition's chronic nature of IBS, coupled with its varying manifestations from one individual to another, underscores the challenge of managing it through a singular approach. This complexity necessitates a comprehensive strategy that addresses the wide array of factors contributing to the disorder. The introduction of such diverse methodologies not only caters to the physical aspects of IBS but also considers the psychological, dietary, and lifestyle dimensions that play critical roles in the overall wellbeing of those affected. Dietary adjustments play a crucial role in managing IBS, with strategies such as the Low-FODMAP Diet offering significant relief for many. This diet highlights the importance of personalized nutrition in managing the condition.

The Low-FODMAP Diet

FODMAPs, an acronym for Fermentable Oligosaccharides, Disaccharides, Monosaccharides, And Polyols, represent a group of short-chain carbohydrates that are poorly absorbed in the small intestine. These compounds, naturally found in a wide array of foods, have drawn significant attention in nutritional science and gastroenterology for their role in digestive health.

FODMAPs encompass several types of carbohydrates that, due to their structure and how they are processed in the gut, can be difficult for some people to digest. Oligosaccharides are found in foods like wheat, rye, legumes, and various fruits and vegetables. Disaccharides, with lactose being the most prominent member of this group, are present in dairy products. Monosaccharides, notably fructose, are abundant in fruits, honey, and high-fructose corn syrup. Polyols, sugar alcohols like sorbitol and mannitol, are found in certain fruits and vegetables and are also used as artificial sweeteners.

Each of these carbohydrates can contribute to digestive discomfort in sensitive individuals, largely due to their fermentation by gut bacteria and their osmotic effect, which draws water into the gut.

The link between FODMAPs and digestive symptoms arises from two primary mechanisms: the osmotic effect and fermentation.

The first one occurs when FODMAPs, being poorly absorbed in the small intestine, draw water into the intestinal lumen. This increase in water can lead to diarrhea in susceptible individuals, contributing to the urgency and frequency of bowel movements associated with IBS. Fermentation, on the other hand, takes place when the undigested FODMAPs reach the large intestine, where they become substrates for gut bacteria. The fermentation process produces gas, which can lead to bloating, distension, and abdominal discomfort. Furthermore, the rapid fermentation of FODMAPs can alter gut motility, exacerbating symptoms of both diarrhea and constipation.

The collective impact of these mechanisms makes FODMAPs a significant dietary consideration for individuals with IBS and similar functional gastrointestinal disorders. The variability in individual tolerance to different FODMAPs highlights the complexity of their role in digestive health. While some individuals may react strongly to oligosaccharides or lactose, others may find that their symptoms are triggered by fructose or polyols. This variability necessitates a personalized approach to dietary management, one that considers the unique sensitivities and nutritional needs of each individual.

Research into the role of FODMAPs in digestive health has led to the development of the Low-FODMAP Diet, a dietary strategy that reduces the intake of these fermentable carbohydrates. Clinical trials and nutritional studies have demonstrated the efficacy of this diet in managing symptoms of IBS, including bloating, gas, abdominal pain, diarrhea, and constipation. By systematically reducing the intake of high-FODMAP foods and gradually reintroducing them to identify personal triggers, individuals can gain better control over their digestive symptoms.

The Low-FODMAP Diet finds its origins in the groundbreaking research conducted at Monash University in Australia. Developed by a team of gastroenterologists and dietitians, this diet specifically targets the reduction of dietary intake of fermentable carbohydrates. The scientific journey that led to the development of the Low-FODMAP Diet was driven by a deepening understanding of the role these carbohydrates play in digestive health and the management of IBS symptoms.

The genesis of the Low-FODMAP Diet was marked by a series of clinical studies and trials aimed at exploring the relationship between certain carbohydrates and digestive distress. Researchers identified that foods high in FODMAPs could worsen symptoms of IBS. The studies conducted by the Monash team provided empirical evidence supporting the hypothesis that reducing the intake of these fermentable carbohydrates could significantly alleviate these symptoms.

By limiting the intake of high-FODMAP foods, the diet reduces the volume of fermentable substrates available to gut bacteria, thereby decreasing gas production and its associated discomfort. Additionally, the reduction in osmotic activity helps to normalize water content in the intestines, alleviating diarrhea and promoting more regular bowel movements. This dual action—reducing both the osmotic load and the fermentative processes in the gut—underpins the diet's effectiveness in managing IBS symptoms.

Phase One: Elimination

The elimination phase is the initial step of the Low-FODMAP Diet, typically lasting from 2 to 6 weeks. During this period, all high-FODMAP foods are removed from the diet. This includes a wide range of foods that contain the fermentable carbohydrates identified as potential triggers for digestive symptoms. Foods such as certain fruits and vegetables, dairy products with lactose, grains like wheat and rye, legumes, and various sweeteners are excluded.

The primary purpose of this phase is to provide the digestive system with a "reset," allowing for a reduction in symptoms by minimizing the fermentation process in the gut that can lead to gas, bloating, and other IBS-related issues. For many individuals, this phase brings about significant relief from symptoms, serving as an indicator that FODMAPs may be contributing to their digestive discomfort.

During the elimination phase, it is crucial to maintain a balanced diet, ensuring that nutritional needs are met despite the restrictions. This often requires careful planning and, in some cases, the supplementation of certain nutrients to prevent deficiencies.

Phase Two: Reintroduction

Following the elimination phase, the reintroduction phase begins, usually extending over 6 to 8 weeks. This phase involves gradually reintroducing high-FODMAP foods back into the diet one group at a time, allowing the individual to monitor their symptoms and identify which specific FODMAPs trigger their symptoms. This is a meticulous process, where each group of FODMAPs (oligosaccharides, disaccharides, monosaccharides, and polyols) is tested separately by introducing one food from each group at a time and observing the body's response.

The reintroduction phase is critical for identifying personal sensitivities and understanding how different foods impact symptoms. It is during this phase that individuals learn the threshold levels of FODMAPs they can tolerate, which is essential for the development of a personalized diet that balances symptom management with nutritional variety and adequacy.

Phase Three: Personalization

The final phase of the Low-FODMAP Diet is personalization, where the insights gained from the reintroduction phase are used to create a tailored eating plan. This phase focuses on integrating a broader range of foods into the diet while managing symptoms effectively. The goal is to establish a long-term dietary pattern that is both enjoyable and sustainable, avoiding unnecessary restrictions that can lead to nutritional deficiencies and impact quality of life.

During the personalization phase, individuals can enjoy a more varied diet, incorporating many of the foods they love, within the tolerance levels identified in the reintroduction phase. It is also a time for ongoing monitoring and adjustment, as tolerance to FODMAPs can change over time, and dietary flexibility may increase.

Implementing the Low-FODMAP Diet through these three phases offers a structured, evidence-based approach to managing gastrointestinal symptoms associated with FODMAP sensitivity. By systematically eliminating, reintroducing, and personalizing dietary choices, individuals can achieve symptom relief while enjoying a nutritionally balanced and satisfying diet. This phased approach empowers individuals with the knowledge and tools to manage their digestive health effectively, enhancing their overall well-being and quality of life.

For those eager to delve deeper into the Low-FODMAP diet, discover delectable and easy-to-prepare recipes that adhere to this dietary approach, and gain a comprehensive understanding of which foods to embrace and which to avoid, I've authored a resource that promises to be an invaluable companion on your journey. "The Low-FODMAP Diet Cookbook," available on Amazon.com, is meticulously crafted to guide you through the dietary management of IBS and other digestive discomforts. This book not only offers a wide array of tasty Low-FODMAP recipes but also provides an exhaustive list of permissible foods alongside those best avoided, making it an essential guide for anyone looking to navigate the Low-FODMAP diet with ease and confidence. Whether you're a culinary novice or a seasoned chef, this cookbook is designed to enrich your dietary experience, ensuring that managing your digestive health is both delicious and straightforward.

SCAN THE QR CODE

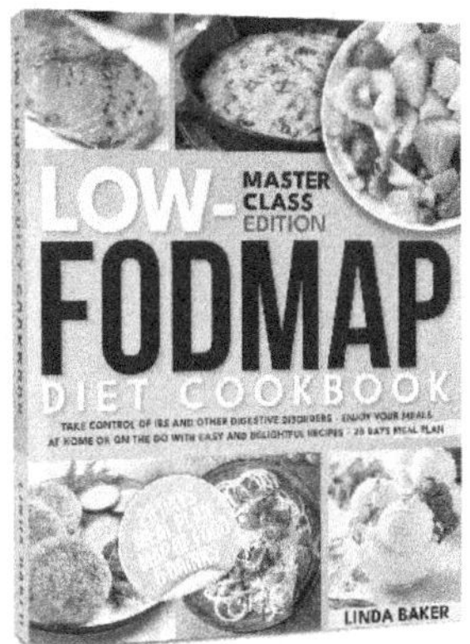

or click this link (eBook only): https://amzn.to/3PdP4ye

Other therapies

Alternative and complementary therapies have gained popularity as adjunctive treatments for managing IBS, offering a holistic approach to alleviating symptoms. These therapies, ranging from herbal treatments and supplements to traditional Chinese medicine practices like acupuncture and the use of natural substances such as peppermint oil, provide diverse options for individuals seeking relief from IBS. It's crucial, however, to approach these therapies with caution and to seek professional guidance to ensure they complement existing treatments safely and effectively.

For instance, herbal treatments and dietary supplements have been explored for their potential benefits. Certain herbs like ginger are known for their gastrointestinal soothing properties, potentially aiding in the reduction of nausea and abdominal discomfort. Another example is slippery elm, which is believed to act as a demulcent, forming a soothing film over the mucous membrane, thereby easing abdominal pain and reducing irritation.

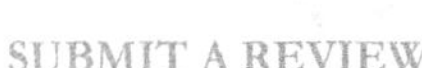

SUBMIT A REVIEW

If you enjoyed this chapter, I would be grateful if you could support me by leaving a review of the book on Amazon. Your feedback is very valuable and inspires me!

It's very simple and only takes a few minutes:

1. Go to the "My Orders" page on Amazon and search for the book "Mind Over Gut".
2. Select "**Write a product review**".
3. Select a Star Rating.
4. Optionally, add text, photos, or videos and select **Submit**.

Chapter 2: How the Brain and Gut Communicate

The communication between the brain and the gut is a complex, two-way street, integral to our overall health and well-being. This dialogue is facilitated by a sophisticated network involving nerves, hormones, and the immune system, ensuring constant interaction between our central nervous system (CNS) and the enteric nervous system (ENS) located in the gut. Understanding this communication requires a dive into the realms of neuroscience and gastroenterology, revealing the intricacies of how these distant parts of our body talk to each other.

At the core of this conversation is the vagus nerve, a critical component of the parasympathetic nervous system, which extends from the brainstem down to the abdomen. Acting as a major highway for information, the vagus nerve transmits signals back and forth between the brain and the gut. For instance, when the brain perceives a threat and triggers a stress response, the vagus nerve can convey this message to the gut, often resulting in a change in gastrointestinal function. This can explain why we sometimes experience stomach discomfort during periods of stress or anxiety.

The Brain-Gut Axis

The exploration of the relationship between gut health and mental well-being evolved over centuries, deeply rooted in the annals of medical history. The ancient Greeks, including the philosopher Hippocrates, often regarded as the father of medicine, posited that all disease begins in the gut. This early intuition hinted at the profound impact of gastrointestinal health on the overall well-being of an individual, setting the stage for millennia of inquiry and discovery.

As we traverse through history, the 19th and early 20th centuries marked a period of burgeoning interest in the connections between diet, digestion, and mental health. Physicians and scientists of the era observed and documented cases where alterations in the digestive system seemed to influence mood and cognitive functions, suggesting a complex interplay between the mind and the gut. However, these observations were often sidelined by the dominant biomedical models that prioritized the brain as the sole organ of interest in matters of mental health.

The concept of the brain-gut axis as we understand it today began to take a more definitive shape with the advent of modern science and technology, allowing for a deeper investigation into how these two systems communicate. This axis is defined by the bidirectional communication network that links the emotional and cognitive centers of the brain with peripheral intestinal functions. This network encompasses various pathways, including the central nervous system (CNS), the enteric nervous system (ENS), the autonomic nervous system (ANS), the hypothalamic-pituitary-adrenal (HPA) axis, and the complex signaling mechanisms involving neurotransmitters, hormones, and immune system molecules.

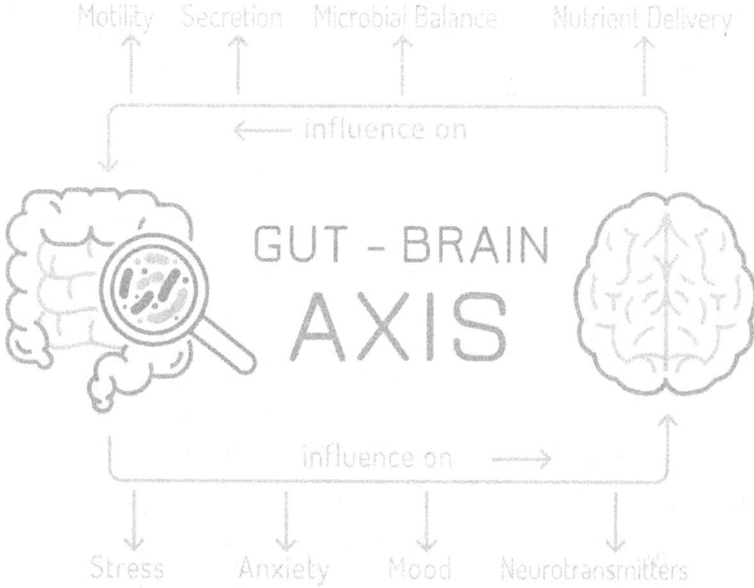

Research has shown that the diverse community of microorganisms residing in the gut can produce neurotransmitters, interact with the immune system, and influence the barrier function of the intestines, thereby affecting brain health and mood. This gut microbiota's ability to communicate with the brain through these various pathways has opened new horizons in understanding the etiology of mental health disorders and their potential treatments. Environmental factors, such as diet, stress, and antibiotics, can significantly impact the composition of the gut microbiota and, consequently, the communication between the gut and the brain.

The historical perspective on gut health and mental well-being, coupled with the contemporary definition of the brain-gut axis, provides a comprehensive framework for understanding this complex relationship. It highlights the importance of considering both the gut and the brain in the quest for optimal health, reflecting a paradigm shift in how we approach mental and physical health issues. This evolving understanding encourages a more integrated and nuanced approach to healthcare, where the ancient wisdom that "all disease begins in the gut" finds its modern scientific validation in the study of the brain-gut axis.

The Science of the Second Brain

The concept of the "second brain" might sound like a figure of speech, yet it encapsulates a profound truth about the human body that science has only begun to unravel in recent decades. This second brain, known scientifically as the enteric nervous system (ENS), resides within the lining of our gastrointestinal tract. Far from being a mere conduit for digestion, the ENS is an intricate network of over 100 million neurons—more than in either the spinal cord or the peripheral nervous system. This remarkable discovery has shifted the way we understand the gut, positioning it as a critical player in our overall health and well-being, especially in its communication with the brain.

The ENS operates with a high level of autonomy from the brain, controlling the processes of digestion, nutrient absorption, and gut motility. Yet, it is in constant communication with the central nervous system (CNS), influencing and being influenced by our mental state. This bi-directional communication occurs through a variety of pathways, including the nervous system, hormonal signals, and the immune system, highlighting the complexity and significance of the brain-gut axis.

One of the most striking aspects of the gut's role in this communication network is its production of serotonin, a neurotransmitter often associated with feelings of happiness and well-being, which we will focus on in the following paragraphs.

The science of the second brain, with its focus on the ENS, neurotransmitters, and the gut's role in serotonin production, provides a compelling glimpse into the interconnectedness of our body's systems, highlighting the holistic nature of health and the importance of nurturing our gut as much as our brain. It suggests that maintaining a healthy gut is not just about physical health but is also intrinsically linked to our mental and emotional well-being.

Serotonin

Serotonin is a neurotransmitter synthesized in the brain and the gastrointestinal tract, which influences a wide array of bodily functions, demonstrating the interconnectivity of mental and physical health.

Serotonin is perhaps best known for its impact on mood and emotions. It contributes to feelings of happiness and well-being, and its balance is critical for emotional stability. The brain's serotonergic system, which involves the pathways through which serotonin signals are transmitted, is a focal point in the study of psychiatric disorders, including depression and anxiety. Serotonin's role in these conditions is underscored by the action of selective serotonin reuptake inhibitors (SSRIs), a class of medications that work by increasing the availability of serotonin in the brain, thereby alleviating symptoms of depression and anxiety. This therapeutic effect highlights the direct link between serotonin levels and mood regulation.

Beyond its influence on mental health, serotonin exerts a powerful effect on the body's appetite and digestive functions. It is involved in regulating hunger and satiety signals, playing a key role in food intake and eating behaviors. Serotonin's presence in the gastrointestinal tract, where approximately 95% of the body's serotonin is found, underscores its importance in digestion. It regulates bowel movements and gut motility, ensuring the proper functioning of the digestive system. By modulating the contraction of smooth muscle in the intestines, serotonin facilitates the movement of food along the digestive tract, affecting the speed at which digestion occurs and influencing overall gut health.

The relationship between serotonin and digestion extends to the neurotransmitter's role in gut-brain communication where the gut-brain axis is influenced by serotonin levels. This connection illustrates how digestive processes can impact mental well-being and vice versa. For instance, alterations in gut serotonin levels can lead to changes in gut motility and function, which may contribute to gastrointestinal disorders such IBS. Conversely, psychological stress can affect serotonin signaling in the gut, further demonstrating the interconnectedness of emotional states and digestive health.

Serotonin's wide-ranging effects on the body highlight its importance also as a signaling molecule that bridges the gap between the brain and the gut. Its role in regulating mood, appetite, and digestion exemplifies the complexity of the body's internal communication networks and the delicate balance required for maintaining health. The study of serotonin and its functions continues to shed light on the mechanisms underlying the interplay between mental and physical health, offering potential pathways for therapeutic interventions in both psychiatric and gastrointestinal disorders.

Microbiota and Mental Health

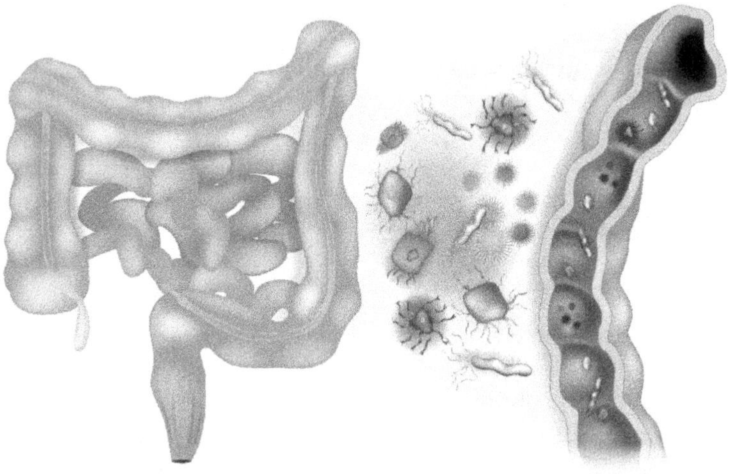

As seen in the previous paragraphs, the gut microbiota plays a crucial role, weaving together the threads of physical well-being and mental health. This complex community of microorganisms, comprising bacteria, viruses, fungi, and protozoa, resides within our gastrointestinal tract and performs functions that affect the body far beyond the confines of digestion. The gut microbiota influences everything from nutrient absorption and immune function to the production of vitamins and neurotransmitters.

Each person's microbiota is unique, shaped by factors such as diet, lifestyle, and exposure to antibiotics.

Through the brain-gut axis, bacteria can send signals to the brain, influencing brain function and, consequently, affecting mood and cognition. These microorganisms produce a variety of neuroactive substances, including neurotransmitters and metabolic by-products, that can impact brain health. For example, certain strains of bacteria are known to produce gamma-aminobutyric acid (GABA), a neurotransmitter that helps regulate feelings of anxiety and stress.

The balance of our gut microbiota is delicate, and when this equilibrium is disrupted—a condition known as dysbiosis—the consequences can extend to our mental health. Dysbiosis has been associated with a range of mood and cognitive disorders, including depression, anxiety, and even autism spectrum disorders. The mechanisms behind these effects are multifaceted, involving changes in neurotransmitter production, increased inflammation, and alterations in the gut barrier function, which may allow harmful substances to enter the bloodstream and potentially reach the brain.

Furthermore, the impact of dysbiosis on mood and cognition underscores the importance of a healthy gut microbiota for mental well-being. Studies have shown that probiotics, which are beneficial bacteria, can have positive effects, suggesting that interventions targeting the gut microbiota could offer new avenues for treating mood disorders. This research highlights the potential of modulating the gut microbiota as a means of influencing brain health, pointing to diet, probiotic supplementation, and lifestyle changes as tools for maintaining physical health and emotional well-being.

Stress and the Gut-Brain Dialogue

The relationship between stress and the gastrointestinal system is a prime example of how closely the brain and gut communicate. This network involves various bodily systems that respond to psychological stress, impacting gut function and health. Understanding this interaction requires delving into the physiological mechanisms at play, the consequences of stress on the gut, and how different coping strategies can influence gut health.

When faced with stress, the body activates its stress response system, involving both the central nervous system and the endocrine system. This response is designed to prepare the body to confront or flee from perceived threats, a primal reaction that has physiological effects on various organs, including the gut. Stress can alter gut motility—the way the gut moves food along—change the secretion levels of digestive juices, and even affect the permeability of the gut lining. These alterations are the body's attempt to prioritize resources in response to stress, but when stress is chronic, they can lead to gastrointestinal discomfort and dysfunction.

Chronic stress is particularly problematic for the gut. It can disrupt the normal balance and function of the gut microbiota, the production of certain vitamins, and even neurotransmitters. Stress can increase intestinal permeability allowing bacteria and toxins to pass into the bloodstream and trigger inflammation. This state of affairs can contribute to or worsen conditions such as IBS, IBD, and gastroesophageal reflux disease (GERD), highlighting the need for effective stress management to maintain gut health.

Addressing the impact of stress on the gut involves employing various coping mechanisms and lifestyle changes. Physical activity, for instance, can reduce stress levels and improve gut motility and microbiota composition. Mindfulness and meditation practices have been shown to lower stress and may positively affect gut health by reducing inflammation and improving the integrity of the gut barrier. Diet also plays a significant role; eating a balanced diet rich in fiber, probiotics, and prebiotics can support a healthy gut microbiota, which in turn can enhance resilience to stress.

In addition to lifestyle modifications, psychological therapies like cognitive-behavioral therapy (CBT) can be effective in managing stress. These therapies work by changing patterns of thinking and behavior that contribute to stress, thereby reducing its physiological impact on the gut. Stress management techniques, such as relaxation training and biofeedback, offer additional tools for individuals to control their stress responses, potentially mitigating the adverse effects on gut health.

Moreover, hypnosis, which will be discussed in this book, can also help with managing the impact of stress on the gut. We will learn more about its role and benefits in the following chapters, further exploring how this therapeutic approach can complement other strategies to support gut health and overall well-being.

Nutrition's Role in the Brain-Gut Connection

The role of nutrition in the brain-gut connection underscores the adage "you are what you eat," highlighting how diet directly influences our mental and physical health through its impact on the gut microbiota and the brain.

Dietary choices play a pivotal role in shaping the gut microbiota.

A diet rich in varied and whole foods, particularly those high in fiber such as fruits, vegetables, and whole grains, can promote a diverse and healthy microbiota. This diversity is very important because a well-balanced gut microbiota supports efficient digestion, nutrient absorption, a strong immune system, and a reduced risk of chronic diseases. Fiber acts as a prebiotic, feeding beneficial gut bacteria and enabling them to produce short-chain fatty acids (SCFAs), compounds that have been shown to strengthen the gut barrier, reduce inflammation, and even influence mood and cognitive functions through the gut-brain axis.

Nutrients that specifically benefit the brain and gut include omega-3 fatty acids, found in fatty fish, flaxseeds, and walnuts; these fats are essential for brain health, aiding in the maintenance of neuron function and reducing inflammation. Antioxidants, present in berries, nuts, and green leafy vegetables, combat oxidative stress in both the brain and gut, protecting cells from damage. Probiotic foods like yogurt, kefir, and fermented vegetables introduce beneficial bacteria to the gut, supporting a healthy microbiota balance that is essential for both gut health and mood regulation.

Conversely, the impact of processed foods and additives on the brain-gut connection is increasingly recognized as detrimental. High consumption of processed foods, which are often low in fiber and high in sugar, fat, and artificial additives, can lead to dysbiosis. Moreover, additives found in processed foods, such as emulsifiers and artificial sweeteners, have been shown to disrupt the microbiota and negatively affect mood and cognitive functions, further illustrating the intricate relationship between diet, the gut microbiota, and brain health.

Gut Instincts and Decision-Making

As seen, the "second brain" communicates directly with the brain via the vagus nerve, transmitting signals that can affect emotional and cognitive centers. These signals are not just simple, reflexive responses to hunger or satiety but carry information about the gut's internal environment, which can influence mood, motivation, and decision-making.

Psychological theories provide further insight into how gut feelings operate within the decision-making process. One such theory is the somatic marker hypothesis, proposed by neuroscientist Antonio Damasio. It suggests that emotional processes guide (or bias) behavior, particularly decision-making, through the association of certain physical sensations (somatic markers) with past outcomes. These markers are bodily states that arise from the emotional evaluation of an action's consequences, and they are felt as gut feelings. According to this theory, these somatic markers are crucial for quick and effective decision-making, especially in complex and uncertain situations where rational analysis alone may fall short.

Moreover, the concept of embodied cognition, another psychological theory, supports the idea that our cognitive processes are deeply rooted in the body's interactions with the environment. This theory suggests that the brain is not the sole operator of cognition; rather, cognitive processes are influenced by the body's physical interactions with the world, including those stemming from the gut. Thus, gut feelings can be understood as a form of embodied knowledge, providing intuitive insights that influence decision-making beyond conscious reasoning.

"Hypnotherapy has been a game-changer for me, going beyond what I ever imagined. Before, I avoided eating out and opted for takeaways, eating alone at home. Car rides with anyone but my husband or son were a no-go, and even simple pleasures like getting my nails done felt overwhelming, making me feel trapped. But now, here I am, enjoying a deluxe pedicure — something I couldn't have fathomed doing before my hypnotherapy journey. It's incredible!"

Chapter 3: The Power of Hypnosis

In the preceding chapters, we delved into the intricacies of IBS, unveiling its common forms, underlying causes, and far-reaching effects. A critical aspect we explored was the important role of the brain-gut axis, revealing how the dynamic communication between the brain and the gastrointestinal system profoundly influences both our physical and mental well-being. As we transition into this chapter, our focus shifts toward an innovative and promising therapeutic approach: hypnosis. This exploration aims to illuminate how hypnosis, with its profound benefits, seamlessly integrates with other strategies to manage stress's impact on the gut, bolster its health, and enhance overall well-being. Our journey into the realm of hypnotherapy serves as an introductory guide to its application as a treatment modality for IBS, laying a foundation for understanding its therapeutic potential.

Hypnosis, often misunderstood and shrouded in mystery, is a state of focused attention, enhanced suggestibility, and heightened imagination. Contrary to the common portrayal in media as a form of entertainment, clinical hypnosis is a rigorous therapeutic technique. It leverages the mind's ability to influence bodily functions and sensations, making it a potent tool in managing a variety of health conditions, notably IBS. The essence of hypnotherapy lies in its capacity to modulate the brain-gut axis, the bidirectional communication pathway that links the central nervous system and the gastrointestinal system. By engaging this axis, hypnosis addresses both the physical symptoms of IBS and the psychological stressors that exacerbate them, offering a holistic approach to treatment.

The therapeutic journey of hypnotherapy for IBS begins with the practitioner guiding the patient into a deeply relaxed state. In this state, the individual's mind becomes more open to positive suggestions and imagery, aimed at modulating gut function and reducing sensitivity to pain. These suggestions often involve visualizing the digestive system working smoothly or imagining a journey through the body to promote healing and comfort. The scientific rationale behind this approach lies in its capacity to alter the perception of pain and discomfort associated with IBS, thereby diminishing the intensity of symptoms.

Moreover, hypnosis extends its benefits beyond symptom relief, tackling the often-overlooked aspect of stress, a known trigger for IBS flare-ups. By promoting relaxation and stress reduction, hypnotherapy enhances the resilience of the gut against stressors, thereby mitigating their adverse effects. This aspect is crucial, considering the intricate relationship between stress and the worsening of IBS symptoms. Through techniques that foster a state of calm and relaxation, hypnotherapy strengthens the gut's defense mechanisms, contributing to sustained well-being.

Integrating hypnotherapy with other management strategies for IBS further amplifies its benefits. Dietary adjustments, physical activity, and other psychological therapies can work in concert with hypnotherapy, creating a comprehensive treatment plan tailored to the individual's needs. This multifaceted approach addresses the physical aspects of IBS but also the emotional and psychological factors, offering a path to holistic healing.

Imagine hypnotherapy as a gentle guide, leading you through a landscape of relaxation and focused attention. It's like being guided through a serene forest, where each step brings you closer to understanding and easing your body's response to the key exacerbators of IBS symptoms – stress and pain. Here, in the safe space of the subconscious, positive suggestions are planted like seeds, slowly growing to transform your body's response to these challenges.

Addressing Common Concerns and Misconceptions

When discussing hypnotherapy, particularly in the context of IBS management, it's crucial to address and debunk common myths that often surround the practice of hypnosis. These misconceptions can create barriers to treatment, preventing individuals from accessing a potentially life-altering therapy.

One prevalent myth is that hypnosis is akin to mind control or brainwashing. In reality, hypnotherapy is a collaborative process between therapist and patient. It's only about guiding individuals into a state of focused attention and heightened suggestibility to facilitate positive changes in behavior and perception, not about controlling their thoughts or actions.

Another common misunderstanding is that people under hypnosis are asleep or unconscious. Contrary to this, individuals in a hypnotic state are typically very aware and focused. They're in a state of deep relaxation, but their mind remains alert and receptive to suggestions.

There's also a misconception that hypnotherapy is a quick-fix solution. While many people experience significant benefits from hypnotherapy, it's not a magical cure. Success in treatment often requires multiple sessions and a commitment to practice techniques learned in therapy, such as self-hypnosis and relaxation exercises. Some people believe that only certain individuals are susceptible to hypnosis. However, most people can be hypnotized to some degree. The effectiveness of hypnosis depends more on the individual's openness to the process and willingness to engage with the therapeutic techniques.

The notion that hypnotherapy is unscientific or lacks empirical support is another myth to dispel. Numerous studies have shown the efficacy of hypnotherapy in managing various conditions, including IBS. It's also crucial to understand that hypnotherapy is not a substitute for medical treatment. While it can be an effective complementary therapy for IBS, individuals should continue to follow medical advice and treatment plans as prescribed by their healthcare providers.

Fundamentals of Hypnotherapy

Delving into the essence of hypnotherapy, we uncover a fascinating journey that merges the ancient art of healing with modern psychological insights, revealing the human mind's extraordinary power to initiate self-transformation. Hypnotherapy, often veiled in mystique and clouded by myriad myths, is grounded on a solid foundation of scientific inquiry and psychological understanding. It's akin to embarking on an expedition into our own consciousness, navigating through tranquil waters to uncover the submerged treasures of our subconscious mind. This exploration is not just about psychological renovation but also about appreciating our physiological capabilities, which are frequently underestimated yet profoundly influential.

Let me share with you, from my personal journey, how hypnotherapy stands as a beacon of transformation. Imagine yourself in a state of deep relaxation, akin to floating on a serene, undisturbed lake. This tranquility is what hypnotherapy seeks to achieve—a trance-like state where the hustle and bustle of the conscious mind simmer down, allowing the depths of the subconscious to emerge. This state is not about losing consciousness or falling asleep; quite the opposite. It's about entering a heightened state of awareness where every sense is amplified, akin to turning up the volume on your surroundings, making everything around you appear more vivid, focused, and within grasp. This heightened awareness paves the way for the therapeutic process, setting the stage for profound and lasting change.

The trance state in hypnotherapy can be likened to an orchestra reaching its peak, guided by a conductor—here, the hypnotherapist—who uses a blend of relaxation and visualization techniques to achieve this crescendo.

This state of focused concentration provides the therapist with a canvas, allowing them to paint strokes of change that bypass the often rigid defenses of the conscious mind to speak directly to the subconscious. This part of our mind, a reservoir of our deepest beliefs, emotions, and patterns, becomes receptive to new ideas and positive suggestions.

One of the cornerstones of this transformative journey is guided imagery.

Drawing from my own experiences, I recall vividly how this technique was used to address my struggles with IBS. The therapist guided me through a peaceful visualization of my digestive system working in perfect harmony, a journey that brought significant relief from the discomfort and anxiety that had become all too familiar. This is just one example of how hypnotherapy employs vivid, positive imagery to evoke physical and emotional responses that align with healing and well-being.

Another crucial aspect is suggestion therapy, where the therapist integrates positive suggestions into the subconscious. These suggestions are like seeds sown in fertile soil, designed to blossom into healthier thoughts, emotions, and behaviors after the session. It's a process that underscores the collaborative nature of the therapeutic relationship, one built on trust, rapport, and a shared vision for the outcome of therapy.

This therapeutic alliance is the golden thread that ties the hypnotherapist and client together, a partnership founded on mutual respect and a deep understanding of the individual's unique psychological landscape. The therapist's ability to tailor the therapy to the individual's needs is paramount, creating a bespoke journey of transformation.

Beyond the confines of the therapy room, hypnotherapy empowers individuals to take control of their healing journey. It teaches the art of self-hypnosis, a skill that enables continued progress and self-management, especially vital for those dealing with chronic conditions like IBS. This empowerment aspect is what sets hypnotherapy apart, offering a long-term tools for managing symptoms and enhancing quality of life.

The Physiological State of Relaxation through Hypnosis

The physiological state of relaxation achieved through hypnosis is a fascinating and complex process that significantly diverges from ordinary rest or sleep. This state, often characterized by an altered level of consciousness, shifts the individual's focus away from external stimuli and internal worries, directing attention inward to a state of calm and balance.

Central to the physiological relaxation induced by hypnosis is the significant reduction in the activity of the sympathetic nervous system (SNS), the branch of the autonomic nervous system responsible for the "fight or flight" response. This response is characterized by an increase in heart rate, blood pressure, and muscle tension, preparing the body to respond to perceived threats. Hypnosis counters this response by activating the parasympathetic nervous system (PNS), often referred to as the "rest and digest" system. This activation leads to a decrease in heart rate, a lowering of blood pressure, and a relaxation of muscle tension, signaling the body to enter a state of rest and recuperation.

The transition from sympathetic to parasympathetic dominance under hypnosis has profound effects on the body's physiological processes. For example, breathing becomes slower and deeper, promoting oxygenation of the blood and facilitating a sense of physical relaxation. Muscle tension decreases, alleviating pain and discomfort associated with chronic stress and anxiety. Additionally, this shift towards parasympathetic activation aids in regulating digestive processes, which can be adversely affected by stress and anxiety, illustrating the interconnectedness of the relaxation state induced by hypnosis with the body's physical health. Moreover, the state of relaxation achieved through hypnosis has a direct impact on the brain's neurochemistry. Studies have shown that hypnosis can influence the release of serotonin and dopamine.

Neurobiological Changes under Hypnosis

Neuroimaging studies, particularly those utilizing functional magnetic resonance imaging (fMRI) and positron emission tomography (PET), have been instrumental in identifying the brain regions and networks involved in hypnosis. These studies reveal that this state leads to distinct changes in brain activity, with notable alterations observed in the prefrontal cortex, anterior cingulate cortex, thalamus, and default mode network (DMN). The prefrontal cortex, associated with higher-order cognitive processes and executive functions, shows increased activation, suggesting a heightened state of focused attention and cognitive control during hypnosis. Conversely, the DMN, typically active during mind-wandering and self-referential thoughts, exhibits decreased activity, indicating a reduction in self-consciousness and a shift away from habitual mental patterns.

Counteracting Stress Responses through Hypnosis

The stress response is a complex physiological and psychological reaction to perceived threats and challenges. While this response is essential for survival, chronic activation due to prolonged stress can lead to a myriad of health issues, including anxiety, depression, hypertension, and weakened immune function. Hypnosis, through its capacity to induce deep relaxation and alter mental states, offers a promising avenue for mitigating the adverse effects of stress on the body and mind.

Case Studies, Research and Efficacy of Hypnotherapy

The exploration of hypnotherapy's effectiveness in treating IBS has been a subject of considerable research. Multiple studies have underscored the significant role hypnotherapy can play in alleviating IBS symptoms. These research efforts, rigorous in methodology and expansive in scope, provide compelling evidence supporting hypnotherapy as a viable treatment option for IBS.

Clinical trials have consistently shown that hypnotherapy can lead to marked improvements in the primary symptoms of IBS, including abdominal pain, bloating, and bowel irregularities. Notably, these improvements are often long-lasting, with many patients reporting sustained relief well beyond the treatment period. This enduring effect suggests that hypnotherapy may induce deep-rooted changes in how the body processes and responds to IBS triggers.

Moreover, research indicates that the benefits of hypnotherapy extend beyond physical symptom relief. Patients undergoing hypnotherapy have reported enhanced quality of life, reduced anxiety and depression levels, and improved psychological well-being.

The mechanisms behind hypnotherapy's success in treating IBS are thought to involve the modulation of the gut-brain axis. By calming the mind and inducing a state of relaxation, hypnotherapy can mitigate the stress responses. Furthermore, the cognitive aspects of hypnotherapy, such as reframing pain perception and fostering a positive mindset, play a crucial role in its effectiveness.

Despite these promising findings, hypnotherapy remains underutilized in the management of IBS, often overshadowed by more conventional treatments. This underutilization may stem from misconceptions about hypnotherapy or a lack of awareness about its proven benefits. However, as awareness grows and more healthcare professionals embrace this approach, hypnotherapy is poised to become an integral part of IBS treatment plans.

A study found in the Journal of Crohn's and Colitis (2021), provides a comprehensive evaluation of the effectiveness of gut-directed hypnotherapy compared to standard medical treatment (SMT) in managing IBS-type symptoms in patients with quiescent Inflammatory Bowel Disease (IBD).

The study's methodology included a multicentre randomized controlled open-label trial. A total of 80 patients, aged 12-65 years with an established diagnosis of Crohn's disease or ulcerative colitis and in clinical remission, were included. These patients were randomly allocated to either hypnotherapy or SMT, with treatments spanning over 12 weeks, followed by a follow-up phase up to 40 weeks.

The hypnotherapy protocol was detailed, involving six sessions over 12 weeks, focusing on exercises for general relaxation, stress control, control of abdominal pain, gut and immune functioning, and improving self-esteem. The sessions were adapted to each participant's specific issues. In contrast, SMT involved sessions at the outpatient clinic, offering various modalities like dietary advice, medications, and lifestyle adjustments.

The primary outcome measure was a reduction of $\geq 50\%$ on the Irritable

Bowel Syndrome Severity Scoring System (IBS-SSS) at week 40 compared to baseline. Secondary outcomes included total IBS-SSS score, quality of life, adequate relief, IBS-related cognitions, and depression and anxiety scores.

The results showed no significant difference in the primary outcome between the two groups. Nine patients in each group (27% in SMT and 30% in hypnotherapy) met the primary outcome. The study also observed similar adequate relief rates and secondary outcomes between the two groups.

The study concluded that while hypnotherapy was not superior to SMT, both treatments were reasonable options for managing IBS-type symptoms in IBD patients in remission. It suggested that the choice of treatment might depend on the patient's preference and individual clinical scenario.

Another study by V. Miller (Neurogastroenterology Unit, Wythenshawe Hospital, Manchester, UK), H. R. Carruthers (Neurogastroenterology Unit, Wythenshawe Hospital, Manchester, UK), J. Morris (Department of Medical Statistics, Wythenshawe Hospital, Manchester, UK.), S. S. Hasan (Hypnotherapy Unit, Wythenshawe Hospital, Manchester, UK), S. Archbold (Neurogastroenterology Unit, Wythenshawe Hospital, Manchester, UK), and P. J. Whorwell (Neurogastroenterology Unit, Wythenshawe Hospital, Manchester, UK), presents a compelling narrative about the effectiveness of gut-focused hypnotherapy for patients with refractory IBS. This extensive study involved a large cohort of 1,000 patients, predominantly female, aged between 17 and 91 years, who had not responded to conventional treatments. The age range and gender distribution are significant as they reflect the typical demographic most affected by IBS, underscoring the relevance and applicability of the study findings to a broad patient population.

The treatment approach adopted in this study was gut-focused hypnotherapy, delivered by a team of trained therapists. This specific form of hypnotherapy is noteworthy as it emphasizes gaining control over the gastrointestinal system, an aspect often disregarded in traditional medical treatments for IBS. The therapy consisted of an initial consultation followed by several hypnotherapy sessions. Each session was tailored to the individual's symptoms and was designed to teach them how to exert control over their gut functions. This patient-centric approach is crucial in the context of IBS, a condition characterized by a wide variety of symptoms that can vary greatly from person to person.

The study's outcome measures were centered around the IBS Symptom Severity Score, a widely recognized tool for assessing the severity of IBS symptoms. The findings were remarkable, with a significant proportion of patients (76%) experiencing a clinically significant reduction (50 points or more) in their IBS-SSS following three months of hypnotherapy. This level of response is noteworthy, particularly considering the refractory nature of the patient population. Furthermore, the study employed stricter criteria for improvement, and even under these conditions, a substantial proportion of patients showed notable improvements in their symptom scores.

Beyond the primary symptoms of IBS, the study also observed improvements in related psychological aspects, such as anxiety and depression. This is a critical finding, as these mental health conditions are often comorbid with IBS and can exacerbate the physical symptoms. Additionally, the study reported improvements in noncolonic symptoms like lethargy and backache, which are frequently reported by IBS patients but are not always directly addressed in treatment.

One of the most significant implications of this study is its demonstration of the wide-ranging benefits of hypnotherapy. It highlights that hypnotherapy is not only effective in improving the core symptoms of IBS but also enhances the overall quality of life for patients.

SUBMIT A REVIEW

If you enjoyed this chapter, I would be grateful if you could support me by leaving a review of the book on Amazon. Your feedback is very valuable and inspires me!

It's very simple and only takes a few minutes:

1. Go to the "My Orders" page on Amazon and search for the book "Mind Over Gut".
2. Select "**Write a product review**".
3. Select a Star Rating.
4. Optionally, add text, photos, or videos and select **Submit**.

Chapter 4: Hypnotherapy Sessions

When considering hypnotherapy, it's vital to approach it with realistic expectations, understanding both its potential and its limits. Hypnotherapy is not a panacea; it's a therapeutic tool that requires time, patience, and active engagement. One of the first steps is understanding that changes through hypnotherapy can be gradual. The therapy works on influencing the subconscious mind, a process that varies widely among individuals. For some, relief from symptoms might be swift and profound, while others may experience a more subtle or gradual improvement. Patience here is not just a virtue but a necessity.

Hypnotherapy is most effective when integrated into a comprehensive IBS management plan, which might include dietary adjustments, medication, and other stress management techniques. Hypnotherapy is particularly adept at managing symptoms like pain and discomfort, as well as reducing stress and anxiety. However, expecting it to entirely eradicate IBS can lead to disappointment, at least that was the case for me.

Setting clear, achievable goals is key to a successful hypnotherapy experience.

These goals should reflect personal health objectives, whether it's reducing the severity of symptoms, improving digestive function, or enhancing overall well-being. Having specific aims helps to track progress, provides motivation, and brings a sense of accomplishment as these goals are gradually met.

Entering hypnotherapy with a balanced view of its possibilities and limitations helps create a more fulfilling and effective therapeutic experience. It's about aligning expectations with reality, preparing for a journey that may have ups and downs, but ultimately leads to a better understanding and management of IBS. This approach fosters a mindset ready for the gradual yet impactful changes that hypnotherapy can bring.

Choosing a Qualified Hypnotherapist

Selecting a qualified hypnotherapist is a critical decision in your journey towards managing IBS. The effectiveness of hypnotherapy largely depends on the expertise and approach of the practitioner. It's essential to choose a hypnotherapist who is not only well-trained and experienced in hypnotherapy but also familiar with treating gastrointestinal disorders like IBS.

Seek out professionals with credible certifications in hypnotherapy from recognized institutions. Additionally, look for practitioners who have a background in healthcare or psychology, as they often bring a deeper understanding of the interconnectedness of physical and mental health.

Before deciding, consider arranging a preliminary consultation. This meeting provides an opportunity to discuss your specific case of IBS, understand their approach to treatment, and gauge whether their style aligns with your comfort and needs. A good hypnotherapist should make you feel at ease, listen attentively to your concerns, and clearly explain the hypnotherapy process.

Remember, the rapport between you and your hypnotherapist is crucial for a successful therapeutic experience, so choose someone with whom you feel a sense of trust and comfort.

Hypnosis Techniques

In a typical hypnotherapy session, the therapist may start by guiding you into a relaxed state using deep breathing and muscle relaxation techniques. Once a state of calm is achieved, the therapist introduces guided imagery tailored to your symptoms and experiences. This process is not merely about reaching a temporary state of relaxation but about engaging deeply with techniques that have the potential to alter your relationship with your body and its response to stress.

As we delve deeper into the subsequent paragraphs, we will explore in detail the intricacies of these relaxation and guided imagery techniques. We will have a comprehensive overview of the benefits these practices offer, not just in the realm of physical symptoms but also in the broader context of mental and emotional well-being. We'll examine the scientific underpinnings that make these techniques effective, shedding light on how they can induce changes in the body's stress response, potentially alleviating the discomfort and distress associated with IBS.

Moreover, we'll offer practical insights into how these methods can be seamlessly integrated into your daily routine, empowering you with tools to manage symptoms and enhance your quality of life. From understanding the step-by-step process of progressive muscle relaxation to exploring the transformative power of guided imagery and soothing sound therapy, we aim to provide a holistic view of how hypnotherapy can offer relief and support for those navigating the complexities of IBS.

Deep breathing

Deep breathing, often known as abdominal or belly breathing, is a fundamental technique focusing on full and rhythmic inhalations and exhalations. It is especially useful in hypnosis and serves as an excellent foundational practice for beginners in breathing techniques. This technique engages the diaphragm, a large muscle at the base of the lungs. As you breathe in deeply, the diaphragm contracts and moves downward, enabling the lungs to expand and fill with air. This action increases oxygen intake and stimulates the parasympathetic nervous system, or the 'rest and digest' system, leading to a relaxation response in the body.

The relevance of deep breathing in hypnosis for IBS is significant due to several reasons. Firstly, it triggers the body's relaxation response, shifting from the stress response to a more relaxed state, crucial in managing IBS symptoms that often worsen due to stress. Secondly, it enhances the mind-body connection, allowing individuals to become more attuned to their bodily sensations, which is essential in hypnotherapy for effective treatment. Furthermore, deep breathing helps in reducing stress and anxiety, common triggers or aggravators of IBS symptoms.

Suggestion Therapy

Suggestion therapy taps into the power of your subconscious mind to positively influence and improve your IBS symptoms and overall experience. This technique is based on the understanding that your mind can directly affect your physical health, suggesting that changing your thought patterns can lead to significant improvements in gut function. During a typical session of suggestion therapy, a hypnotherapist will help you enter a deeply relaxed state. Once you're in this state of heightened suggestibility, your therapist will introduce carefully designed positive affirmations and suggestions.

For example, the therapist might suggest that your gut is becoming calmer and more regulated, or that you are becoming more resilient to the triggers of IBS. These suggestions are potent tools that can modify the neural pathways responsible for the stress and pain responses associated with IBS. Once your subconscious mind becomes open to these positive affirmations, it can start a healing and adjustment process within your body.

The advantages of suggestion therapy go beyond the sessions themselves. You can learn self-hypnosis techniques, enabling you to continually reinforce these positive suggestions in your daily life. This empowerment is essential for managing a chronic condition like IBS, giving you the tools to take control of your symptoms.

Progressive Muscle Relaxation (PMR)

Progressive Muscle Relaxation is a relaxation technique that involves the deliberate tensing and then relaxing of different muscle groups throughout the body. This method is particularly beneficial for IBS relief, as stress and tension are known to worsening the symptoms of this condition.

The principle behind PMR is simple yet profound. By systematically working through the body, tensing each muscle group firmly but not to the point of strain, and then releasing the tension, individuals can achieve a deep state of physical relaxation.

Whether lying down or sitting in a chair with feet planted firmly on the ground, the goal is to ensure that the body is in a state conducive to relaxation. Initiating the relaxation process involves deep breathing exercises, focusing on slow inhalations through the nose followed by exhalations through the mouth, setting a foundational calm for the body.

As the core of PMR lies in the tension and relaxation of muscle groups, the technique involves a systematic approach. Starting from the lower extremities, such as the feet, and moving upwards through the body to the facial muscles, each muscle group is tensed for approximately five seconds before being released. This act of tension, followed by immediate relaxation, allows for a stark contrast in sensations, fostering a deeper understanding and appreciation of the body's state of relaxation.

For instance, tensing the muscles in the feet and calves by curling the toes downwards or tightening the thigh muscles can highlight areas of the body that typically hold stress. The deliberate act of releasing this tension, coupled with focused breathing, can lead to a profound sense of physical relaxation. This journey through the body continues, encompassing the arms, hands, shoulders, neck, and even the facial muscles, ensuring that no area is neglected.

Soothing Sound Therapy

Soothing Sound Therapy harnesses the gentle power of calming sounds or music to enhance relaxation techniques, offering a complementary tool for hypnotherapy. The auditory environment plays a pivotal role in facilitating deep relaxation and mental tranquility, making it a valuable ally in the quest for well-being.

Our sensory experiences, particularly what we hear, can significantly influence our emotional and physiological states. Nature sounds, such as the rhythmic crashing of ocean waves, the soft patter of rain, or the tranquil whisper of a forest breeze, have a natural harmony that many find inherently calming. Similarly, soft instrumental music, with its gentle harmonies and melodies, can provide a serene backdrop that supports relaxation practices and guided imagery, creating an auditory space conducive to mental and physical relaxation.

Guided Imagery and Relaxation

Guided imagery and relaxation involve taking you through vivid, calming mental images and scenarios, significantly impacting your body's physiological responses, especially in the digestive system. Guided imagery centers on creating mental pictures that bring about peace and well-being. For you this might mean visualizing a tranquil environment or picturing your digestive system functioning smoothly and without pain. Such mental imagery stimulates the same neural pathways as real-life experiences, affecting bodily functions that the subconscious mind controls, like gut motility and sensitivity.

Relaxation techniques enhance guided imagery by easing stress and tension throughout your body. These techniques may include deep breathing exercises, progressive muscle relaxation, or mindfulness meditation. They assist in transitioning your body from a state of stress (sympathetic activation) to one of calm (parasympathetic activation). This relaxation response can lessen gut hypersensitivity, diminish inflammation, and normalize gut movements, directly tackling the physical symptoms of IBS.

The real value of guided imagery and relaxation is in their adaptability. You can tailor the imagery to fit your own experiences and goals, making the approach more effective and engaging. Furthermore, you can practice these techniques outside of therapy sessions, through self-hypnosis or recorded guides, offering a handy tool for continuous symptom management.

Self-Hypnosis

Self-hypnosis involves learning to enter a state of deep relaxation and focused attention, where you can apply therapeutic suggestions and visualizations on your own. Once you're relaxed, you can use pre-learned scripts or affirmations targeting specific IBS symptoms or stressors. For example, you might focus on visualizing your digestive system functioning smoothly or affirming your ability to stay calm and relaxed even when IBS symptoms arise.

The beauty of self-hypnosis lies in its flexibility and accessibility. You can practice it at your convenience, making it an ideal tool for daily stress management and symptom control. It becomes your personal sanctuary, a means to reclaim control over your body's reactions to IBS triggers.

Moreover, self-hypnosis can be tailored to your unique experience with IBS. Through self-exploration, you can identify the most effective imagery and affirmations for your situation. This personalization makes self-hypnosis an incredibly effective tool in the long-term management of IBS.

If you're new to self-hypnosis, it's advisable to initially work with a qualified hypnotherapist who can guide the learning process and provide personalized scripts. As your proficiency grows, you can adapt and create your own scripts, further enhancing the effectiveness of this self-managed approach.

Incorporating self-hypnosis into your daily routine can also reinforce the benefits achieved in formal hypnotherapy sessions. It acts as a continuous support system, providing relief and stability even outside the therapist's office.

SUBMIT A REVIEW

If you enjoyed this chapter, I would be grateful if you could support me by leaving a review of the book on Amazon. Your feedback is very valuable and inspires me!

It's very simple and only takes a few minutes:

1. Go to the "My Orders" page on Amazon and search for the book "Mind Over Gut".
2. Select "**Write a product review**".
3. Select a Star Rating.
4. Optionally, add text, photos, or videos and select **Submit**.

Chapter 5: Real-Life Stories

As I embarked on this illuminating journey to explore the realms of, I found myself delving into a world far richer and more complex than I had initially imagined. This exploration was not confined to clinical studies or medical journals but extended into the realm of personal experiences and heartfelt narratives. These stories, which form the crux of this chapter, emerged from a series of group sessions dedicated to hypnotherapy that I attended on the recommendation of a psychologist.

These sessions were more than just meetings; they were confluences of resilience, determination, and hope. Here, I met a diverse group of individuals, each with a unique story to tell about their battle with IBS. These were not mere anecdotes but testimonies of real people who had faced the turmoil of IBS and emerged stronger. They shared how their journey with IBS was not solely confined to dietary adjustments like the Low-FODMAP diet. Instead, it was a more holistic approach where hypnotherapy played a very important role.

In these sessions, I witnessed remarkable tales of transformation. Many participants had mastered their condition, turning their struggles into a source of strength. This mastery was not an overnight miracle but the result of relentless perseverance and an unwavering commitment to change. Some of them spoke about how hypnotherapy opened doors to self-awareness and control, allowing them to view IBS not as a life sentence but as a manageable aspect of their lives.

The change in these individuals was not just psychological but also manifested in their lifestyles. They adopted various strategies and tools, some as simple as daily relaxation techniques, others as complex as a complete overhaul of their routines and habits. These changes were not just about alleviating physical symptoms but also about reclaiming the joy and spontaneity of life that IBS had once overshadowed.

During these enriching sessions, I also had the opportunity to engage with numerous professionals and doctors specializing in IBS and hypnotherapy. Their insights added a new dimension to my understanding, bridging the gap between clinical expertise and personal experiences. The professionals highlighted the significance of a tailored approach in hypnotherapy, one that addresses the unique nuances of each individual's experience with IBS.

As I share these stories in the following paragraphs, it is my hope that they serve as beacons of hope and guidance. Each story is a testament to the power of resilience and the potential of hypnotherapy in transforming lives affected by IBS. Through these narratives, we uncover the challenges, celebrate the successes, and most importantly, learn from the journeys of those who have walked the path before us.

Emily's First Hypnotherapy Session Changed Her Life

Emily is a 38-year-old graphic designer who found her life persistently overshadowed by the relentless grip of IBS. The condition had become an uninvited guest, turning everyday activities into a minefield of anxiety and discomfort. The constant fear of an unexpected flare-up, the cramping, and the unpredictability of her symptoms kept her on edge, impacting her work and straining her relationship with her family.

> *"The day started with a challenge. Waking up with that familiar unease in my stomach, I knew it would be one of those days. The cramps, the urgency - it's like an invisible chain holding me back. I hesitated before my morning coffee, remembering my doctor's advice about potential triggers."*

It was during a particularly challenging phase, riddled with discomfort and despair, that Emily stumbled upon a forum discussing the benefits of hypnotherapy. Skeptical yet desperate for relief, she delved deeper into the stories shared by others who had found solace in this unconventional approach. The accounts of transformation intrigued her, igniting a flicker of hope in her weary heart. Compelled by these stories, Emily scheduled her first hypnotherapy session. The initial meeting with her hypnotherapist was a profound experience. She was introduced to the concept of the gut-brain connection, a revelation that reshaped her understanding of IBS. The therapist explained how stress and anxiety could worsen her symptoms, triggering her gut's hypersensitivity. This insight was a turning point for Emily, as she began to comprehend the intricate relationship between her mind and her digestive system.

> *"Work was a struggle. The discomfort was a constant distraction, making it hard to concentrate. But I managed, taking deep breaths and recalling the calming techniques from my last session. It's empowering, really, to have these tools at my disposal."*

Guided by her therapist, she learned relaxation techniques and visualization exercises. She would close her eyes and imagine her digestive system functioning smoothly, free from the turmoil that had plagued her for so long. The therapist's soothing voice would guide her through serene landscapes, each session bringing her closer to harmony within her body.

> *"The most significant change I've noticed since starting*

hypnotherapy isn't just in symptom reduction, though that's
substantial. It's the shift in my emotional state - from feeling
victimized by my body to collaborating with it. I'm learning to
listen to it, to understand its signals, and respond with kindness
and care."

Emily started practicing self-hypnosis at home, armed with the knowledge and techniques imparted by her therapist. She dedicated time each day to this practice, finding a quiet corner where she could focus on her breathing and visualize a calm digestive system. These moments of self-hypnosis became her sanctuary, a space where she could exert control over her body's rebellious nature.

"Tonight, I'll do my self-hypnosis session before bed. It's become a
cherished ritual, a space where I nurture hope and healing. Each
session is a step closer to a life where IBS doesn't dictate my
choices."

With each passing day, Emily noticed significant improvements. The frequency and intensity of her IBS symptoms began to diminish. The once overwhelming anxiety started to recede, replaced by a sense of control and empowerment. She felt a growing confidence, not just in managing her symptoms but in her overall approach to life. Encouraged by her progress, Emily integrated lifestyle changes suggested by her therapist. She tweaked her diet, avoiding foods that triggered her symptoms. Mindfulness became a part of her daily routine, helping her stay centered and calm. Yoga, with its focus on breath and body awareness, complemented her hypnotherapy sessions, enhancing her journey towards wellness.

"Reflecting on my journey, I'm grateful for the path of
hypnotherapy. It hasn't been easy, and there are still tough days,
but the progress is undeniable."

Emily's story is a testament to the power of the mind-body connection and the potential of hypnotherapy in managing IBS. Her journey from skepticism to empowerment highlights the profound impact this therapy can have on individuals struggling with this challenging condition. Through her experience, Emily discovered that with understanding, practice, and perseverance, it is possible to find balance and peace even amidst life's uncertainties.

Robert, a Self-Learner about Hypnosis

Robert is a 45-year-old high school teacher. He had his life rhythm disrupted by the nagging symptoms of IBS. For years, he grappled with the condition, which manifested in frequent abdominal pain, discomfort, and the ever-present anxiety about when the next episode would strike. These symptoms made teaching, a job he once loved, a daily challenge, often forcing him to step out of the classroom at the most inopportune moments.

"As a high school teacher, my days are often unpredictable and stressful, which can exacerbate my IBS symptoms."

The turning point came when Robert's colleague mentioned hypnotherapy as a potential treatment for IBS. Initially skeptical, Robert's curiosity got the better of him, and he began researching. The more he read, the more he realized that this could be the key to regaining control over his life. One evening, while searching for alternative IBS treatments, Robert came across an article on self-hypnosis. Intrigued, he delved deeper, reading extensively about the mind-gut connection and how self-hypnosis could help in managing IBS symptoms. He decided to take a self-reliant approach to his condition.

Robert started his journey by purchasing some relaxation CDs. He would listen to them every night, focusing on the soothing melodies and guided imagery designed to relax the mind and, in turn, the gut. This routine became an integral part of his evenings, slowly bringing a sense of calm to his life.

Encouraged by the initial relief, Robert began exploring more about self-hypnosis. He read books and online resources, learning techniques to deepen his relaxation and visualization skills. He practiced these techniques diligently, visualizing a calm and functional digestive system, free from the turmoil of IBS.

"Focusing on my breathing and visualizing a calm, functioning digestive system, I felt a tangible release of tension."

As weeks turned into months, Robert noticed a significant improvement in his symptoms. The abdominal pain and discomfort became less frequent, and his anxiety levels dropped. He felt a newfound sense of control over his body, a feeling that had eluded him for years.

Robert's self-guided journey with hypnotherapy marked a turning point in his life. He regained his confidence and joy in teaching, no longer hindered by the fear of an IBS episode.

Robert's journey with self-hypnosis and IBS stands as a powerful illustration of how knowledge, dedication, and self-care can significantly alter one's experience with this challenging condition. His story unfolds as a compelling narrative of self-discovery where he learns to tune into his body's signals, understanding and managing his symptoms through the practice of self-hypnosis.

> *"The self-hypnosis techniques I've been practicing have become a*
> *powerful tool in my arsenal against IBS. Whenever I felt a hint*
> *of discomfort, I would discreetly use my relaxation techniques,*
> *drawing on the affirmations and visualizations that resonate with*
> *me."*

This approach transformed his life, demonstrating the remarkable potential of self-guided techniques in providing relief and restoring control. Robert's experience is a beacon of hope, showing that with the right tools and a commitment to self-care, living well with IBS is within reach.

Interviews with Hypnotherapy Practitioners and Patients

These interviews are an invaluable resource, providing a comprehensive understanding of hypnotherapy's role in managing IBS. From the practitioners' viewpoint, interviews often delve into their professional journey into specializing in hypnotherapy for IBS, their therapeutic approaches, and the philosophies underpinning their practice. They share insights into the nuances of treating IBS with hypnotherapy, discussing techniques such as guided imagery, suggestion therapy, and self-hypnosis. Practitioners also reflect on the challenges and rewards of their work, including patient success stories and the intricacies of tailoring therapy to individual needs.

In contrast, interviews with patients provide a window into the lived experience of IBS and its treatment through hypnotherapy. Patients discuss their initial skepticism or hopes about hypnotherapy, their journey through the treatment process, and the outcomes they've experienced. They offer first-hand accounts of how hypnotherapy has impacted their symptoms, daily life, and overall well-being. These narratives often touch on the emotional and psychological aspects of living with IBS, including the struggles of dealing with a chronic, often misunderstood condition.

These interviews also address common misconceptions and barriers to seeking hypnotherapy. Practitioners and patients alike share their thoughts on why hypnotherapy might be overlooked as a treatment option and what can be done to increase its acceptance and accessibility. They discuss the importance of patient education, the need for empathy in treatment, and the role of ongoing support in managing a chronic condition like IBS.

Moreover, these interviews explore the evolving landscape of hypnotherapy. Practitioners may discuss recent advancements, ongoing research, and future prospects for hypnotherapy in the broader context of IBS treatment. Patients, on the other hand, might share their insights on living with IBS in a changing world, including adapting to new treatments and maintaining long-term symptom management.

The names of the hypnotherapists have been intentionally omitted, and the initials used are entirely fictitious. This choice reflects my belief that selecting a hypnotherapist should be a personal decision, free from external influences. The rapport with your therapist is crucial, built on trust and respect. Therefore, it's essential to communicate openly and choose a therapist whose personality and approach align closely with your own.

Interview with Dr. J. H., Hypnotherapist Specializing in IBS Treatment

Linda: Dr. H., thank you for joining us. Could you start by telling us about your approach to treating IBS with hypnotherapy?

J. H.: Absolutely. My approach to hypnotherapy for IBS is grounded in scientific understanding and tailored to individual needs. The gut-brain axis plays a crucial role in IBS, and hypnotherapy effectively addresses this connection. By guiding patients through specific mental imagery and suggestion techniques, we can influence gut function and alleviate IBS symptoms.

Linda: Fascinating. Could you share some details about the techniques you used with Emily, one of your patients?

J. H.: Certainly. Emily came to me with typical IBS symptoms: chronic abdominal pain and discomfort. During our sessions, I focused on gut-directed hypnotherapy. This involved guided imagery where Emily visualized her digestive system functioning smoothly and without pain. We used specific suggestions to promote gut relaxation and normalize bowel movements.

Linda: How did Emily respond to these techniques?

J. H.: Emily responded remarkably well. Initially, she was a bit skeptical, but as we progressed, she became more receptive. The key was her willingness to engage deeply with the visualization exercises. She reported a significant reduction in her symptoms after just a few sessions.

Linda: That's impressive. What kind of suggestions did you give her for self-hypnosis?

J. H.: For self-hypnosis, I encouraged Emily to focus on positive affirmations about her gut health. I suggested she visualize a calm, peaceful gut environment every day. We also worked on stress-reduction techniques, as stress is a known trigger for IBS symptoms.

Linda: In light of your extensive experience, what would you say are the main benefits of hypnotherapy for IBS?

J. H.: Hypnotherapy offers a non-invasive, effective way to manage IBS symptoms. It empowers patients to take control of their condition through mind-body techniques. Additionally, it often leads to improved overall well-being, not just relief from IBS symptoms.

Reflecting on Dr. J. H.' insightful interview, it's clear that the scientific underpinnings of hypnotherapy are crucial in treating IBS effectively. The way Dr. J. H. described Emily's treatment showcases a methodical and evidence-based approach, aligning perfectly with contemporary research on the gut-brain axis. His emphasis on individualized therapy, grounded in scientific understanding, not only validates the therapeutic process but also echoes the growing body of research underscoring hypnotherapy's efficacy. This interview, combined with Emily's remarkable progress, offers compelling evidence of how a scientifically informed approach to hypnotherapy can lead to substantial improvements in managing IBS symptoms.

Interview with Dr. M. R., Expert in IBS Diet and Holistic Approaches

Linda: Dr. M. R., thank you for joining us today. Could you start by sharing your perspective on IBS, its causes, and symptoms?

Dr. M.R.: Thank you, Linda. IBS is a complex syndrome that impacts the large intestine, leading to symptoms like abdominal pain, bloating, gas, diarrhea, and constipation. While the exact causes are still being unraveled, it's clear that factors like diet, stress, and gut-brain interactions play pivotal roles.

Linda: Dr. M.R., can you elaborate on the dietary approach for managing IBS? What specific changes do you recommend?

Dr. M.R.: Certainly, Linda. Dietary management in IBS often involves identifying and reducing foods that trigger symptoms. This can vary from person to person, but common irritants include high-FODMAP foods, dairy, and gluten. We start by eliminating these potential triggers and then gradually reintroduce them to identify specific sensitivities. It's a tailored approach, ensuring that patients don't unnecessarily restrict their diet.

Linda: How do you ensure patients maintain a balanced diet while following these restrictions?

Dr. M.R.: That's a critical aspect. We work closely with dietitians to ensure that while certain foods are eliminated or reduced, the overall diet remains nutritionally balanced. This might involve introducing alternative sources of fiber, vitamins, and minerals to compensate for the removed items.

Linda: What about patients who struggle with dietary changes?

Dr. M.R.: Behavioral and motivational strategies are key here. We encourage small, gradual changes rather than drastic alterations. Also, educating patients about the impact of diet on IBS symptoms can be a significant motivator for them to adhere to dietary recommendations.

Linda: Interesting. Speaking of gut-brain interactions, how do you incorporate hypnotherapy into your treatment approach alongside diet?

Dr. M.R.: Great question. While diet modification is essential for managing IBS, I've found that integrating hypnotherapy can be profoundly effective. It addresses the psychological and emotional dimensions of IBS. Stress reduction and mental well-being are crucial in alleviating symptoms, and hypnotherapy directly targets these aspects.

Linda: Have you seen significant improvements in your patients who combine diet changes with hypnotherapy?

Dr. M.R.: Absolutely. Patients who engage in both dietary management and hypnotherapy often report better symptom control, improved quality of life, and reduced anxiety related to their IBS. It's a holistic approach that acknowledges the multifaceted nature of IBS.

Linda: Lastly, what would you say to someone hesitant about trying hypnotherapy for IBS?

Dr. M.R.: I'd encourage them to keep an open mind. Hypnotherapy, particularly when combined with dietary adjustments, can provide relief that might not be achieved through traditional methods alone. It's a safe, non-invasive approach that can make a real difference in managing IBS.

Reflecting on Dr. M.R.' interview, it's evident that integrating dietary strategies with hypnotherapy offers a comprehensive approach to managing IBS. His insights into dietary modifications underscore the importance of a balanced, personalized diet in alleviating IBS symptoms. Moreover, Dr. M.R.' advocacy for hypnotherapy as a complementary treatment highlights the significance of addressing both physical and psychological factors in IBS management. This harmonious blend of diet and hypnotherapy, as suggested by Dr. M.R., resonates with the holistic perspective that I advocate for in managing IBS, ensuring a multifaceted approach to this complex condition.

Chapter 6: Practical Exercises

Disclaimer

In advocating for the pursuit of hypnotherapy as a means to alleviate IBS symptoms, my primary recommendation is to consult a professional hypnotherapist. They are uniquely equipped to navigate you through the intricacies of this therapeutic journey towards relief. However, if you're inclined to initially explore the potential benefits and foundational concepts on your own, the insights shared in the forthcoming sections are designed to illuminate the path to well-being you might discover through self-guided exploration.

The narrative of individuals who have embarked on a self-taught journey to manage their IBS symptoms is both inspiring and telling. Many have found significant improvement in their condition by diligently applying self-hypnosis techniques and deepening their understanding of the mind-gut connection. This could very well be your experience. Nevertheless, I underscore the value of partnering with an experienced practitioner not because self-guided efforts bear inherent risks, but rather to enhance the efficiency and depth of your learning. A skilled hypnotherapist can expedite your mastery of the necessary skills, ensuring a robust foundation from which to build your self-management strategies.

This chapter aims not just to advocate for professional guidance but also to empower you with knowledge. By familiarizing yourself with the principles and practices detailed here, you'll gain a clearer view of the potential for transformation that hypnotherapy holds. Remember, the journey to managing IBS is as unique as the individuals who embark on it, and whether through guided or self-directed paths, the destination of greater well-being remains the same.

Choose a Quite Room

To practice these exercises effectively, it's essential to select an environment that is tranquil, serene, and comfortable, minimizing distractions to foster a deep connection with your inner self. This concept aligns with what is known in Buddhist practice as the "container principle"—the idea that the setting or context creates conducive external conditions, enabling us to harness and internalize the surrounding active forces for our benefit. The right 'container' might encompass various elements, including furniture, colors, lighting, or natural aspects, all designed to facilitate a reconnection and rejuvenation of our inner essence.

Choosing an ideal location for these exercises is crucial; it should be as quiet as possible. Thus, areas frequented by others or prone to noise from people or pets should be avoided to prevent overstimulation of the senses. Spaces associated with stress, such as an office or home office cluttered with work-related items like papers and desks, are not suitable for practices like self-hypnosis or meditation. Instead, opt for a space where tranquility prevails—perhaps a bedroom, a living room with doors and windows closed, or any area where you feel at ease and confident of undisturbed privacy.

A few additional suggestions for creating the ideal space include embracing minimalism, which helps reduce distractions by limiting the number of items in the room. Consider having just a few essentials, such as a small table, a yoga mat, or large, soft pillows for lying down during rest or meditative practices. Incorporating natural elements can enhance the sense of balance and harmony within the space. While there are no strict guidelines, introducing elements like floral arrangements, possibly with jasmine for its fragrance, vases of flowers, or containers filled with sand and shells, can enrich the environment. For those able, adding a water fountain can provide a sublime touch, replicating the calming presence of nature, particularly beneficial for meditation if practicing by the sea or in natural surroundings isn't feasible.

Creating this peaceful and harmonious setting is crucial for achieving the depth of concentration and relaxation necessary for engaging fully in the hypnotherapy process. This carefully curated ambiance supports a deeper exploration of the self, enhancing the overall effectiveness of your practice.

Breathing Techniques

Begin your practice with brief sessions lasting 2-3 minutes to acquaint yourself with the breathing technique. As you grow more accustomed to the method, extend the duration of your sessions to 5-10 minutes for optimal benefits. Aim to incorporate this practice into your daily routine, ensuring consistency in your efforts. Select a tranquil and cozy setting for your initial practices to minimize distractions and enhance your focus on the breathing process. Should you find your thoughts drifting during the practice, gently redirect your attention to the rhythm of your breath, using it as an anchor to the present moment. Consider integrating these breathing exercises into your hypnotherapy sessions or any relaxation routine to facilitate a smooth transition into a state of deep relaxation, laying a solid foundation for the session ahead.

Alternate-Nostril Breathing

Known also as Nadi Shodhana in traditional yogic practices, alternate-nostril breathing is a calming and balancing "pranayama" that involves alternating the flow of breath through each nostril. This technique is designed to harmonize the two hemispheres of the brain, promote mental clarity, and balance the body's energy channels.

The process begins by sitting in a comfortable, upright position to ensure free flow of breath and energy.

...Settle your left hand comfortably on your lap and position your right hand near your face.

...Using your right hand, place your index and middle fingers at the center of your forehead, just above your eyebrows, using them lightly as a stabilizing point. The thumb and ring finger are the ones you'll be actively using.

...Gently close your eyes and draw a deep breath in and out through your nose.

...Use your right thumb to gently close off your right nostril. Breathe in slowly and deeply through the left nostril.

...Seal your left nostril with your ring finger, so both nostrils are closed, and hold your breath for a short pause at the peak of your inhalation.

...Uncover your right nostril and exhale smoothly through the right side, pausing for a moment after the exhale.

...Take a slow breath in through the right nostril.

...Close off both nostrils again (using your thumb and ring finger).

...Release your left nostril and exhale gently through the left side, pausing momentarily after the exhale.

...Continue for five to 10 cycles, letting your attention follow the flow of your breaths in and out.

4-7-8 Breathing

This breathing technique developed by Dr. Andrew Weil is a simple yet powerful breathing exercise designed to promote relaxation and reduce stress. By extending the length of the exhale relative to the inhale, the technique encourages a reduction in heart rate and blood pressure, fostering a state of calm throughout the body.

Begin by sitting upright with a straight back. After becoming proficient in this breathing technique, you have the option to lie down.

...Position the tip of your tongue against the gum ridge just behind your upper front teeth and maintain this placement throughout the practice.

...Fully exhale from your mouth, producing a whooshing noise.

...With your mouth closed, take a silent inhale through your nose, counting to four in your mind.

...Retain your breath, silently counting up to seven.

...Release your breath through your mouth, again making a whooshing sound, as you count to eight.

Belly Breathing

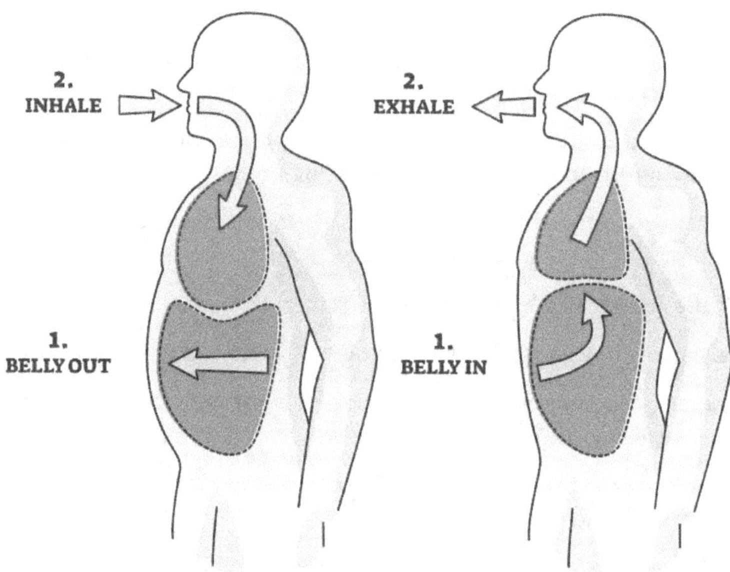

Belly breathing (diaphragmatic breathing or abdominal breathing) is a fundamental breathing technique that focuses on engaging the diaphragm, a large muscle located at the base of the lungs. This technique encourages full oxygen exchange and is known for its ability to reduce stress, lower heart rate and blood pressure, and promote relaxation. It stands in contrast to shallow chest breathing, which can increase tension and anxiety.

In belly breathing, the aim is to consciously breathe deeply into the lungs, causing the belly to rise and fall significantly more than the chest. This method maximizes the amount of oxygen drawn into the body, enhancing overall oxygenation, stimulating the parasympathetic nervous system and fostering a state of calm throughout the body and mind.

Choose a comfortable position, such as sitting upright in a chair, adopting a cross-legged posture, or lying flat on your back with adequate support for your head and knees.

...Rest one hand gently on your chest and place the other just beneath your ribcage on your abdomen.

...Ease your abdomen into a relaxed state, avoiding any intentional tightening or contraction of your muscles.

...Inhale slowly and deeply through your nose, guiding the breath so that it fills your lungs and causes your stomach to expand under your hand, while the hand on your chest should remain mostly motionless.

...Exhale with controlled breath through lips that are slightly puckered, being mindful that the hand on your chest should stay still, indicating minimal movement in the upper chest.

...Repeat this breathing pattern for as many cycles as feels comfortable, starting perhaps with three cycles and increasing the count as you become more familiar with the technique.

Four-Square (Box Breathing)

This technique is a simple yet powerful breathing exercise designed to reduce stress and enhance focus by regulating the breath. This method involves four main steps, each lasting an equal duration, typically four seconds, creating the visual metaphor of a box or square.

...Breathe out for a four-second count.

...Keep your lungs empty, counting to four.

...Draw breath in, timing it to four seconds.

...Retain the breath in your lungs, counting up to four.

...Exhale and restart the sequence.

Panic Breathing

Panic breathing is a potent method specifically designed to counteract panic attacks, facilitating a swift return to calmness. This technique can be exceptionally beneficial in managing sudden episodes of distress, such as during an IBS flare-up when away from the comfort of home. It involves a controlled pattern of breathing that helps stabilize the body's response to stress, effectively calming the nervous system and mitigating the symptoms of panic.

However, caution is advised when employing panic breathing, as it can sometimes lead to dizziness. This is typically a result of the rapid changes in carbon dioxide levels in the blood, which can affect your sense of balance. Therefore, it's crucial to use this technique judiciously—only in moments of acute need—to avoid potential side effects. It's not recommended as a frequent practice but rather as a strategic intervention to manage sudden anxiety or panic attacks.

To ensure safety and maximize the technique's effectiveness, consider practicing panic breathing while seated or in a secure environment where you can safely manage any feelings of lightheadedness that may arise. This mindful approach to panic breathing underscores the importance of using such powerful techniques responsibly, tailoring them to your body's needs and reactions, especially during vulnerable moments like an IBS flare.

...Inhale sharply through the nose in two counts: "1, 2..."

...Do not completely fill the lungs.

...Immediately exhale forcefully through the mouth.

...The entire process should happen quickly.

Progressive Muscle Relaxation

Developed by Dr. Edmund Jacobson in the early 20th century, PMR involves sequentially tensing and then relaxing specific muscle groups throughout the body. This process promotes an awareness of physical sensations associated with relaxation versus tension. This technique not only aids in releasing physical tension but also encourages mental relaxation, making it an effective tool for managing anxiety, stress, and even improving sleep quality.

…Close your eyes gently and take a few deep breaths to start relaxing your body. With each exhale, try to release any tension you're holding.

…Begin with your feet. Tense the muscles in your feet by curling your toes downward as if you are trying to grasp something with them. Hold this tension for a count of 5.

…Now, release the tension in your feet suddenly. Feel the difference in sensation as the muscles relax. Notice the warmth and lightness that follow the release. Pause for 10 to 15 seconds to enjoy the sensation of relaxation.

…Move up to your lower legs. Tense the muscles in your calves by pulling your toes towards you, creating a stretch in your calf muscles. Hold for a count of 5.

…Release the tension and allow your calf muscles to relax. Observe the relaxation spread through your lower legs, soothing and calming the muscles.

Wait for another 10 to 15 seconds, savoring the relaxed state.

...Continue this process with each muscle group in your body, moving upward from your legs to your abdomen, hands, arms, shoulders, neck, and face. For each area, tense the muscles as much as you can (without causing discomfort), hold for a count of 5, and then release the tension suddenly.

...Focus on the contrast between tension and relaxation in each muscle group. This awareness helps deepen the relaxation effect.

...After you have moved through all the muscle groups, spend a few minutes just lying or sitting quietly, breathing deeply and evenly. Enjoy the sense of peace and relaxation that envelops your body.

...When you're ready, open your eyes slowly. Move gently and take a moment to adjust before standing up.

Begin with brief sessions lasting between 5-7 minutes, and as you grow more comfortable with the technique, extend your practice to 15-20 minutes. Incorporate Progressive Muscle Relaxation (PMR) into your daily routine, ideally before bedtime or during periods of increased stress, to aid in anxiety reduction and enhance relaxation. This technique is versatile and can be adapted to alleviate various forms of pain, including headaches and the abdominal discomfort associated with conditions like IBS. When practicing PMR, as you inhale, envision drawing breath into the area of discomfort, and as you exhale, imagine the breath flowing through the painful region, carrying the discomfort away with it. This visualization enhances the PMR technique, promoting a deeper sense of relief and well-being.

Hypnotherapy Script

Induction

Begin by closing your eyes and focusing on your breathing. Take a deep, slow breath in, filling your lungs with calmness. As you exhale, imagine releasing any tension or stress. With each breath, feel yourself becoming more relaxed, more at ease.

Now, visualize yourself standing at the top of a beautiful staircase. This staircase represents your journey into a deeper state of relaxation. Each step is a step closer to peace and healing.

Take the first step down. As your foot touches the step, a wave of relaxation sweeps over you.

Ten... feel your worries drifting away.

Nine... your muscles loosen and relax.

Eight... you're sinking deeper into tranquility.

Seven... each step brings you closer to a state of complete peace.

Six... your mind calms and clears.

Five... halfway there, embraced by a deep sense of relaxation.

As you continue down the staircase,

Four... let go of any remaining tension.

Three... almost at the bottom, feeling completely at ease.

Two... you are surrounded by tranquillity and comfort.

One... you have arrived at a special place of serenity, a safe and peaceful haven created by your mind.

Deepening

Now that you are in your special place of serenity, let's deepen this peaceful state. Imagine a gentle, calming energy radiating from the ground beneath you. With each breath you take, this soothing energy rises up through your body, filling every part of you with a deep sense of calm.

Feel this energy like a warm, comforting light. It starts at your feet, making them heavy and relaxed. It moves slowly up your legs, releasing any tension as it goes. Notice how your knees soften and your thighs let go of their hold.

As this warm energy continues to rise, it soothes your lower back, unwinding any tightness there. Feel it moving up your spine, vertebra by vertebra, leaving a trail of relaxation. Your abdomen and chest become light and free, your breathing becomes deeper and more rhythmic.

Now, the energy reaches your shoulders, a place where we often hold stress. Feel them dropping, becoming loose and relaxed. This calming light travels down your arms to your hands, and then up to your neck, soothing all the muscles there.

Finally, it reaches your head. Feel your facial muscles relax, your jaw unclenches, your eyes soften, and your forehead smoothes out. Every part of you is now deeply relaxed, deeply at ease.

Therapeutic Suggestions

Within this tranquil state, let's focus on your digestive system. Imagine it as a serene river, flowing smoothly through a lush valley. Each curve and bend in the river is easing out, allowing the water to flow freely, without any obstacles or disruptions.

Visualize this river reflecting your digestive process, becoming more balanced and harmonious. Picture the gentle flow easing any discomfort in your abdomen. Each ripple in the water symbolizes the calming of your gut, reducing inflammation and soothing irritation.

Now, think about the foods you consume. Imagine your body accepting these foods with ease, absorbing nutrients and providing you with energy. There is no discomfort or distress, only a sense of nourishment and well-being.

With every breath, reinforce the belief that your digestive system is functioning optimally. You have the power to manage any sensations of discomfort. They are mere ripples on the surface of the river, easily soothed and calmed.

Embrace the feeling of control over your body. You are no longer at the mercy of IBS symptoms. Instead, you are in command, guiding your digestive system to work in harmony with the rest of your body.

Repeat to yourself:

'My digestive system is calm and balanced.'

'I am in control of my body.'

'I embrace health and comfort with every meal.'

As these affirmations echo in your mind, feel a sense of empowerment.

You have the tools and strength to manage your IBS, leading a life full of health and vitality.

Awakening

Now, as our session nears its end, it's time to gently awaken from this deeply relaxed state. With each number I count, feel a renewed sense of energy and clarity, carrying with you the peace and control you've cultivated here.

1.   …Begin to feel a gentle awakening in your toes and feet, a pleasant tingling sensation that signifies renewed vitality.

2.   …This energy moves up to your legs, filling them with strength and stability, preparing you to step forward into your day with confidence.

3.   …Feel this energy continuing to rise, revitalizing your abdomen and digestive system, leaving them calm and harmonious.

4.   …Your chest, arms, and shoulders are infused with this energy, feeling light and free from any burden.

5.   …Finally, the energy reaches your head, your mind clear and alert, eyes feeling refreshed and ready to open.

As I say the final number, you will feel fully awake, yet carrying the tranquillity and control from this session into your daily life.

6.   …Gently open your eyes, feeling completely awake, refreshed, and ready to embrace the day with a sense of peace and empowerment over your IBS. You are calm, you are in control, and you are ready to enjoy every moment of your life.

Closing

As you now sit here, fully awake and revitalized, take a moment to recognize the positive strides you've made today towards your well-being. It's crucial to remember that the sense of control and tranquility you've discovered in this session resides within you, accessible at any moment you require it.

Before we conclude, let's envision your path forward. Imagine yourself consistently applying these techniques, gradually gaining mastery over your IBS symptoms. You're embarking on a transformative journey, with each day edging you closer to enduring ease and equilibrium.

I urge you to reflect on the insights and sensations that emerged during today's session. Let these reflections steer your progress. As we draw this session to a close, carry forward the sense of empowerment and calm you've cultivated, knowing well that you possess the necessary tools to adeptly manage your IBS.

Importantly, during our time together, you may have noticed moments when your gut felt at peace. I encourage you to hold onto that sensation. Memorize how it feels; it's a powerful ally against IBS attacks that often stem from anxieties and fears rather than dietary causes. In such instances, hypnotherapy demonstrates a remarkable efficacy. Remember, this journey is not one you undertake alone, and with each new day, you are fostering greater harmony between your body and mind, leveraging the profound benefits hypnotherapy offers in navigating and mitigating IBS.

SUBMIT A REVIEW

If you enjoyed this chapter, I would be grateful if you could support me by leaving a review of the book on Amazon. Your feedback is very valuable and inspires me!

It's very simple and only takes a few minutes:

1.   Go to the "My Orders" page on Amazon and search for the book "Mind Over Gut".
2.   Select "Write a product review".
3.   Select a Star Rating.
4.   Optionally, add text, photos, or videos and select Submit.

Chapter 7: Beyond the Book

An essential part of continuing the journey is expanding one's knowledge and understanding of the condition and its treatments.

The role of support groups and online communities in managing this condition cannot be overstated. These platforms offer a sense of community, shared experiences, and a wealth of knowledge, making them an invaluable resource for those undergoing hypnotherapy for IBS. Support groups, whether online or in-person, provide a safe space for individuals to share their experiences, struggles, and successes in managing IBS. These groups often consist of fellow IBS sufferers, healthcare professionals, and sometimes, hypnotherapists who offer insights and advice. The communal aspect of these groups is particularly beneficial, as it helps in reducing feelings of isolation and misunderstanding that many with IBS experience.

Online communities, accessible through various social media platforms, forums, and dedicated websites, offer a platform for individuals to connect with a larger, more diverse group of people with similar experiences. These online spaces are particularly useful for those who might not have access to local support groups or prefer the anonymity and convenience of online interaction. They offer a wealth of shared knowledge, personal stories, and practical tips for managing IBS through hypnotherapy and other complementary therapies.

Furthermore, both can be a source of information about the latest research, treatment options, and resources related to IBS and hypnotherapy. Members often share articles, podcast episodes, webinar links, and other educational materials, helping each other stay informed and educated.

These communities also play a crucial role in advocacy and raising awareness about IBS. By sharing their collective experiences, they help in dispelling myths and misconceptions about the condition, promoting a better understanding and more compassionate approach towards those living with IBS. In addition, many of these groups organize events, workshops, and seminars that can be highly beneficial. These events may feature talks from medical professionals, hypnotherapists, nutritionists, and others who specialize in IBS treatment, providing valuable learning opportunities and the chance to ask questions and seek advice.

Continuing Education and Personal Growth

Continuing education is vital in understanding and managing IBS effectively. The field of hypnotherapy and gastrointestinal health is constantly evolving, with new research, techniques, and insights emerging regularly. Staying abreast of these developments can empower individuals to make informed decisions about their treatment and overall health strategy.

Engaging in educational activities, such as attending workshops, seminars, or webinars on IBS and hypnotherapy, can provide valuable information and new perspectives. These events are often led by experts in the field and offer the latest insights into treatment approaches, dietary recommendations, and stress management techniques relevant to IBS.

Reading books, medical journals, and reputable online resources on IBS, hypnotherapy, and related topics is another way to continue one's education. These resources can deepen understanding of the mind-gut connection, the role of stress and diet in IBS, and how hypnotherapy can be integrated with other treatment modalities.

Personal growth is equally important. Living with a chronic condition can be challenging, but it also presents opportunities for growth and self-discovery. Through the process of managing IBS, individuals often develop greater resilience, empathy, and a deeper understanding of their bodies and minds.

Practicing self-reflection and mindfulness can aid in personal growth. Reflecting on one's experiences, challenges, and successes in managing IBS can provide insights into personal strengths and areas for improvement. Mindfulness practices not only aid in symptom management but also promote a greater sense of presence and appreciation for life.

Finally, personal growth involves recognizing and celebrating one's progress, no matter how small. Acknowledging improvements in symptom management, increased knowledge about IBS, or enhanced coping skills reinforces a positive mindset and motivates continued growth and learning.

SUBMIT A REVIEW

If you enjoyed this chapter, I would be grateful if you could support me by leaving a review of the book on Amazon. Your feedback is very valuable and inspires me!

It's very simple and only takes a few minutes:

1. Go to the "My Orders" page on Amazon and search for the book "Mind Over Gut".
2. Select **"Write a product review"**.
3. Select a Star Rating.
4. Optionally, add text, photos, or videos and select **Submit**.

Conclusion

As we draw this book to a close, it's time to reflect on the path we've traversed together. From unraveling the complexities of Irritable Bowel Syndrome to uncovering the transformative power of hypnotherapy, our goal has been to arm you with a wealth of knowledge, actionable strategies, and, most importantly, a renewed sense of hope. IBS, characterized by its multifaceted symptoms and challenges, can profoundly affect one's life. Yet, the exploration of hypnotherapy as a viable treatment avenue unveils promising opportunities for alleviating these symptoms and reclaiming control. By exploring the deep connection between the mind and gut and tapping into the subconscious, hypnotherapy emerges as a distinctive and potent method for IBS management.

Throughout this guide, we've ventured through the scientific underpinnings of hypnosis, the core principles of hypnotherapy, inspiring success stories, and practical advice for incorporating hypnotherapy into your routine. Each section was meticulously designed to not only educate and debunk common misconceptions but also to offer hands-on guidance.

Navigating IBS is a highly individual experience, making this book more than just a source of information—it's a companion on your journey toward better health. It champions ongoing education, heightened self-awareness, and proactive symptom management. Whether you're navigating IBS personally or you're a healthcare provider seeking to enrich your practice, the insights within these pages aim to enlighten, motivate, and support you.

Moreover, this book serves as a testament to the benefits hypnotherapy can offer in the context of IBS. While packed with practical advice and technical insights, it underscores an essential truth: partnering with a therapist remains the most prudent course of action. Hypnotherapy, with its profound capacity to facilitate healing and comfort, can significantly enhance the IBS management strategy when guided by professional expertise. In essence, this guide is a beacon for those looking to understand hypnotherapy's role in IBS treatment, reminding us that the journey to wellness is both a personal and guided endeavor, best navigated with professional support.

About the Author

Linda Baker, a 42-year-old physical education teacher, had navigated the trials of stomach issues from a young age. Despite multiple medical consultations, a resolution to her health problems remained elusive. Consequently, she adapted to her condition, albeit at the cost of the lively social life her peers enjoyed.

Life took a positive turn when, after graduating, Linda met Kevin, her future husband. They married when she was 31, and she became pregnant the following year. During this transformative period, she met Dr. Kim. This skilled physician promptly identified Linda's persistent issue as Irritable Bowel Syndrome and understood the necessity of its management, especially for a smoother pregnancy. Dr. Kim advised Linda to eradicate high-FODMAP foods from her diet, a strategy that significantly improved her health.

With the birth of her second child, Linda found herself challenged by managing family responsibilities, work, and preparing separate meals. However, the quietude of the pandemic period provided her an opportunity to seek practical solutions to harmonize her multifaceted life.

Linda's college education had offered a foundational understanding of the human body. Seeking deeper knowledge, she combined this learning with an array of books and TV cooking shows. This blend of information enabled her to master the Low-FODMAP diet without compromising on taste, and she began sharing these meals with her family, minimizing variations in their dietary routines.

Today, thanks to her diligent studies and lifestyle adjustments, Linda leads a peaceful life. The complaints associated with IBS are largely absent, and she enjoys dining out with friends without the fear of an abrupt departure. Her husband Kevin fully supports her dietary regime, and their children, Sarah (9) and Tom (7), largely follow it as well. Healthy eating has become a family norm, with Linda passionately preparing nutritious meals for them.

Linda's journey with IBS has been a tale of resilience and victory. Over the years, she has used her hard-earned knowledge to assist friends, colleagues, and acquaintances in their battles with IBS. She now seeks to share her experiences more broadly, hoping to enlighten people about the possibility of enjoying life despite IBS through the Low-FODMAP diet and Hypnosis.

www.ingramcontent.com/pod-product-compliance
Lightning Source LLC
Chambersburg PA
CBHW070720260726
48660CB00007B/2660